PEDIATRICS
BOARD
REVIEW

PEDIATRICS
BOARD
REVIEW

Mark Nordness, M.D.

Board Certified Pediatrician
Private Practice
Specialist in Allergy, Asthma, and Immunology
Waukesha Health Care
Milwaukee, Wisconsin

HANLEY & BELFUS, INC.
An Affiliate of Elsevier

The Curtis Center
Independence Square West
Philadelphia, Pennsylvania 19106

Note to the reader: Although the techniques, ideas, and information in this book have been carefully reviewed for correctness, neither the author nor the publisher can accept any legal responsibility for any errors or omissions that may be made. Neither the author nor the publisher makes any guarantee, expressed or implied, with respect to the material contained herein.

Cover photographs: Alexander Withers and Maria Catherine Nordness

Library of Congress Control Number: 2003107049

PEDIATRICS BOARD REVIEW   ISBN 1-56053-584-9

Printed in the United States

Last digit is the print number: 9   8   7   6   5   4   3   2   1

Dedication

This book is dedicated to my parents, Robert and Carole, who taught me the truly important things in life: love, faith, respect, kindness, humility, devotion, and honor.

I also dedicate this book to my loving wife and best friend, Angie, who has been my support and the wind beneath my wings over the many years of my medical training.

Finally, I want to thank my beautiful children, Matthew, Kylie, Michael, Noah and Maria, who remind me every day of the miracles and joys of life.

CONTENTS

PREFACE

Pediatrics Board Review was written to be a succint, fact-based review for newly graduated pediatricians and established pediatricians in preparation for their pediatric board examinations. Now that the recertification examination for board-certified pediatricians has been changed to a "closed-book" exam, there is a need for a review book for busy pediatricians to use in preparation for the examination. This book employs a systems-based approach and covers all the essential information in an easy-to-read format. Key test-taking pearls are included throughout the text.

Although written for pediatricians, medical students would also benefit from the text as a valuable resource during their pediatrics rotation or in preparation for their medical licensing examination.

Mark Nordness, MD

THE ADOLESCENT

Female Birth Control

ESTROGEN/PROGESTERONE PILL

Advantages: Decreased ovarian/endometrial cancer
Reduces menstrual disorders

Disadvantages: Risk of **thromboembolism**
No protection from STDs
Cannot use with breast-feeding

PROGESTIN PILL

Advantage: Can use with breast-feeding

Disadvantages: **Breakthrough bleeding**
No protection from STDs

INJECTABLE AND IMPLANTABLE PROGESTINS

Advantage: Convenience

Disadvantages: Initial irregular menstrual bleeding
Amenorrhea with prolonged use
Minimal weight gain
Hair loss
No protection from STDs
Acne

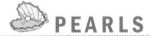 **PEARLS**

Absolute contraindications for the use of hormonal contraceptives include unknown vaginal bleeding, estrogen-dependent tumor, liver disease, thromboembolic disease and cerebrovascular diseases. Relative contraindications are hypertension, migraines, seizures and diabetes mellitus.

Diaphragms and cervical caps are *not recommended* because correct usage requires motivation and comfort inserting the devices. **Intrauterine devices (IUDs)** are *not recommended* for adolescents because of an increased risk of pelvic inflammatory disease.

Drugs of Abuse

COCAINE
- Associated with nasal septal perforation
- Pupils: dilated
- Euphoria, paranoid ideation
- Sympathomimetic: hypertension, tachycardia

ALCOHOL
- Most common **abused drug**
- Pupils: sluggish, normal-sized
- Acute **erosive gastritis** can develop following large ingestions
- Hypoglycemia

MARIJUANA
- Most common **illicit substance** used
- Tachycardia
- Elation
- Euphoria

AMPHETAMINES
- Sympathomimetic: hypertension, tachycardia, hyperactive sweating, tremulousness
- Pupils: dilated

INHALANTS
- Commonly used by younger children
- Associated with **arrhythmias**, renal/liver toxicity and encephalopathy

PHENCYCLIDINE (PCP)
- Sympathomimetic: hypertension, tachycardia
- Cholinergic: diaphoresis, flushing
- **Vertical and horizontal nystagmus**
- Hallucinogenic, **agitation, belligerence**
- Treatment: place patient in quiet room, haloperidol and/or benzodiazepine

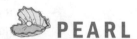 P E A R L

Avoid phenothiazines, because they may cause hypotension.

LSD
- Psychedelic drug
- Sympathomimetic: hypertension, tachycardia and hyperpyrexia
- **Hallucinations** and **acute toxic psychosis**
- Pupils: dilated
- Treatment: place patient in quiet room, haloperidol and/or benzodiazepines

Drugs of Abuse *continued*

GAMMA HYDROXYBUTYRATE

- **"Date rape" drug**
- Central nervous system depressant
- Euphoria
- Overdoses associated with hypotension, bradycardia

ECSTASY

- Used in rave or dance environments
- Relaxation, empathy, **heightened sense of touch**
- Can result in **dehydration**
- Overdoses associated with hypertension, seizures, rhabdomyolysis, acute renal failure or death

Sexually Transmitted Diseases

CHLAMYDIA TRACHOMATIS

Etiology
- *Chlamydia trachomatis*

Presentation
- Females: vaginal discharge (thick cervical discharge)
- Males: dysuria with scant mucopurulent discharge

Diagnosis
- *Chlamydia* inclusion bodies on cell culture, fluorescent antibody, amplification with PCR, DNA probe or enzyme assay

Treatment
- Azithromycin (1 g once) or doxycycline (100 mg BID for 7 days) or erythromycin (500 mg PO QID for 7 days)

Associations
- **Reiter's syndrome**

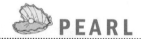

PEARL

Most common **bacterial STD.**

GENITAL WARTS

Etiology
- Human papillomavirus (HPV)

Diagnosis
- Clinical

Treatment
- Cryotherapy, podophyllum or electrocauterization

Risks
- In females, associated with squamous intraepithelial lesions—a precursor for cervical cancer. Must monitor with PAP smears.

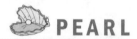

PEARL

Most common **STD** in adolescents in USA.

GONORRHEA

Etiology
- *Neisseria gonorrhoeae* (gram-negative intracellular diplococcus)

Presentation
- Ranges from asymptomatic to purulent discharge (thick cervical discharge)

Sexually Transmitted Diseases *continued*

Complications
- **PID:** involving endometrium/fallopian tubes/peritoneum
- Arthritis (may present with **single joint swelling**/pain)
- **Fitz-Hugh Curtis syndrome** (perihepatitis)
- Endocarditis

Diagnosis
- Culture on Thayer-Martin agar

Treatment
- Ceftriaxone (125 mg IM) or cefixime (400 mg PO) once

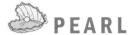

PEARL

Must consider Fitz-Hugh Curtis syndrome in sexually active female with right upper quadrant pain.

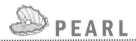

PEARL

Must treat for *C. trachomatis* if treating for gonorrhea.

TRICHOMONAS VAGINALIS

Presentation
- Females: yellow-green frothy malodorous vaginal discharge and **"strawberry cervix"**
- Males: scant clear discharge; usually **asymptomatic**

Diagnosis
- Motile (flagellated) trichomonads on microscopic exam

Treatment
- 2 gm of metronidazole once or 500 mg twice a day for 7 days
- Must treat partner

BACTERIAL VAGINOSIS

Etiology
- *Gardnerella vaginalis*
- Mycoplasmas
- Anaerobic bacteria

Presentation
- Malodorous vaginal discharge

Diagnosis (Need 3 of 4 criteria)
- Vaginal discharge
- pH $\geq$4.5
- positive **"whiff" test** (after KOH added to discharge)
- $\geq$20% clue cells on saline preparation (wet mount)

Risk Factors
- IUD use

Sexually Transmitted Diseases *continued*

BACTERIAL VAGINOSIS *Risk factors continued*

- History of STD
- Smoking
- Uncircumcised male
- Low socioeconomic status

Treatment

- Intravaginal clindamycin or metronidazole cream or PO metronidazole

HERPES

Etiology

- Herpes simplex virus 2/herpes simplex virus 1

Presentation

- **Multiple painful genital ulcers or vesicles**
- Dysuria
- Vaginal/urethral discharge
- Inguinal lymphadenopathy

Diagnosis

- Tzanck smear demonstrates **multinucleated giant cells**
- Culture

Treatment

- Oral acyclovir
  - If started within 6 days of primary infection, decreases viral shedding and new lesion formation
  - Recurrent episode duration can be shortened if acyclovir is started within 2 days of symptoms

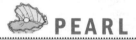 **PEARL**

Untreated, virus can be shed for up to 3 months even if lesions resolve.

SYPHILIS

Etiology

- *Treponema pallidum* (motile spiral organism)

Presentation

- **Painless genital ulcer**
- Inguinal lymphadenopathy

Diagnosis

- RPR, VDRL or FTA-ABS

Treatment

- Benzathine penicillin (2.4 million U IM) or doxycycline (100 mg PO BID) for 14 days

Eating Disorders

BULIMIA NERVOSA

Diagnostic Criteria
1. Recurrent episodes of **binge eating**
2. Fear of not being able to stop eating during binges
3. Regular use of laxatives, vomiting, dieting or fasting
4. Two binge-eating episodes/week for 3 months
5. Body weight/shape determine self-image

Manifestations
- Salivary gland enlargement
- Dental enamel erosion
- Callus over the dorsum of the metacarpophalangeal joints

Treatment
- Psychotherapy, behavior modification and nutritional rehab

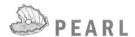

PEARL

Bulimia patients can have normal weights.

ANOREXIA NERVOSA

Diagnostic Criteria
1. Intense **fear of becoming obese**
2. Distorted body image
3. Refusal to maintain minimal body weight for height and age
4. Absence of three consecutive menstrual cycles

Manifestations
- Excessive physical activity
- Preoccupation with food preparation
- Bizarre eating habits
- Often described as "model children"
- **Lanugo, hypothermia, bradyarrhythmias, hypotension**
- Restrictors: severely limit food intake
- Bulimia: binge and purge

Treatment
- Psychotherapy, behavior modification and nutritional rehab

REFERENCES

1. Behrman R, Kliegman R, Jenson H: Nelson Textbook of Pediatrics, 16th edition, Philadelphia, W.B. Saunders, 2000.

2. Tellier P: Club Drugs: Is it all Ecstasy? *Pediatric Annals* 2002;31:550–556.

3. AAP Red Book 2000, 25th edition, 2000.

4. McMillan J, DeAngelis C, Feigin R, Warshaw J: Oski's Pediatrics—Principles and Practice, 3rd edition, Lippincott Williams & Wilkins, 1999.

5. Rudolph C, Rudolph A, Hostetter M, Lister G, Siegel N: Rudolph's Pediatrics, 21st edition, New York, McGraw-Hill, 2002.

ALLERGY

NIH Classification of Asthma

CLASSIFICATION	SYMPTOMS	NIGHTTIME SYMPTOMS	PFTS
Mild intermittent	≤ 2 times/week	≤ 2 times/month	$FEV_1 \geq 80\%$
Mild persistent	> 2 times/week < 1 time/day	> 2 times/month	$FEV_1 \geq 80\%$
Moderate persistent	Daily symptoms Daily use of beta$_2$-agonist Exacerbations affect activity ≥ 2 exacerbations in a week	> 1 time/week	$60\% > FEV_1 > 80\%$
Severe persistent	Continual symptoms Limited physical activity Frequent exacerbations	Frequent	$FEV_1 \leq 60\%$

NIH Stepwise Approach for Treating Asthma in Children Older than 5 Years Old

CLASSIFICATION	QUICK RELIEF	LONG-TERM CONTROL
Mild intermittent	Inhaled beta$_2$-agonist (as needed)	None
Mild persistent	Inhaled beta$_2$-agonist (as needed)	Inhaled corticosteroid (low dose)
Moderate persistent	Inhaled beta$_2$-agonist (as needed)	Inhaled corticosteroid and long-acting beta$_2$-agonist
Severe persistent	Inhaled beta$_2$-agonist (as needed)	Inhaled corticosteroid, long-acting beta$_2$-agonist and oral orticosteroids

NIH Stepwise Approach for Treating Asthma in Children Younger than 5 Years Old

Mild intermittent	Inhaled beta$_2$-agonist (as needed)	None
Mild persistent	Inhaled beta$_2$-agonist (as needed)	Low-dose steroid
Moderate persistent	Inhaled beta$_2$-agonist (as needed)	Inhaled corticosteroid and long-acting beta$_2$-agonist
Severe persistent	Inhaled beta$_2$-agonist (as needed)	Inhaled corticosteroid, long-acting beta$_2$-agonist and oral corticosteroids

Asthma

Manifestations

- Cough with exercise and cold air
- **Nocturnal cough**
- Persistent cough following URI
- Cough with exposure to animals, pollens and cigarette smoke

Diagnosis

- Episodic symptoms of airflow obstruction/ wheezing
- Reversible airflow obstruction
- Change of FEV_1 that is 12% or greater after beta$_2$-agonist

Exercise-Induced Asthma

- Occurs toward the end of exercise;10 minutes after exercise
- Treat 20 minutes before exercise with beta$_2$-agonist
- Occurs in 80% of asthmatics

Medications to Avoid

- Beta-blockers
- Aspirin/NSAID

Reasons for Treatment Failure

- Poor inhaler technique
- Poor compliance
- Environment change

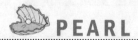 **PEARL**

Psychogenic cough is described as a **brassy/honking cough** that does not occur during sleep.

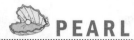 **PEARL**

High concentrations of dust mite exposure in infancy increases the risk of developing asthma.

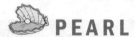 **PEARL**

Nasal polyps are associated with increased incidence of aspirin allergy.

Risks for Asthma Mortality

HOSPITALIZATIONS

- **ICU admissions**
- **Intubation**
- History of sudden severe exacerbations
- Two hospitalizations in the past year
- Three emergency room visits in the past year
- Hospitalization or emergency visit in past month

MEDICATIONS

- Use of **more than two canisters per month** of short-acting inhaled beta$_2$-agonist
- Current use of oral steroids or recent withdrawal from oral steroids

COMPLICATING HEALTH PROBLEMS

- Comorbidity (e.g., cardiovascular disease or COPD)
- Depression or psychosocial problems
- Illicit drug use

OTHERS

- Lack of access to medical care
- *Alternaria* **allergy**
- Poor perception of airflow obstruction or its severity

Theophylline Clearance

DECREASED CLEARANCE WITH INCREASED LEVELS

Disease
- Liver disease
- Congestive heart failure
- Renal failure

Medications
- Erythromycin
- Clarithromycin
- Fluoroquinolones
- Cimetidine
- Ranitidine
- Oral contraceptives
- Ketoconazole
- Propranolol

INCREASED CLEARANCE WITH DECREASED LEVELS

Disease
- Hyperthyroidism
- Cystic fibrosis

Medications
- Carbamazepine
- Phenytoin
- Rifampin
- Phenobarbital

Social Habits
- Smoking

Indications for Venom Immunotherapy

CHILDREN 16 YEARS OLD AND YOUNGER

■ History of **systemic reaction** following sting
- Hypotension
- Wheezing
- Rhinorrhea
- Angioedema
■ **Not indicated** for *only* cutaneous reactions, including pruritus and hives

CHILDREN 17 YEARS OLD AND OLDER

■ History of **systemic reaction** following sting
- Hypotension
- Wheezing
- Rhinorrhea
- Angioedema
■ **Indicated** for cutaneous reactions, including pruritus and hives

Allergic Rhinitis

Risk Factors

- Parental atopy
- Atopic disease (asthma/eczema) with patient

Triggers

SEASONAL

- Spring: tree pollens
- Summer: grass pollens
- Fall: molds/ragweed

PERENNIAL

- Dust mites
- Indoor molds
- Cockroaches
- Cats
- Dogs

Manifestations

- Pale, boggy nasal mucosa
- Extra infraorbital folds **(Dennie-Morgan line)**
- Allergic shiners
- Allergic salute **(nasal crease)**
- High arched palate/dental overbite from mouth breathing

Treatment

- First line—avoidance of allergen
- Second line—intranasal corticosteroid and oral antihistamines
- Third line—immunotherapy if refractory to pharmacotherapy

Food Allergy

Common Foods
- Eggs, wheat, fish, peanut, soy, and milk

Manifestations
- Anaphylaxis
- Gastrointestinal: vomiting, diarrhea, hematochezia, colitis
- Skin: urticaria, angioedema and eczema
- Respiratory: rhinorrhea, cough, sneezing and wheezing

Diagnosis
- **Skin prick testing** (most sensitive method)
- RAST testing (use for severe eczema or dermatographism)

Treatment
- Avoidance

Prevention
- **Breast-feeding** helps delay the development of atopic disease
- Late introduction of highly allergic foods
    - Peanuts, eggs, cow's milk, wheat and soy
    - Helps to delay the onset of atopic disease

Prognosis
- Egg, milk and soy allergies **usually resolve** by 3 years old
- Peanut, tree nut and fish allergies **rarely resolve**

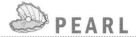 PEARL

Approximately 50% of infants allergic to cow's milk protein have an intolerance to soy protein. Use of a protein hydrolysate formula may be required.

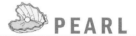 PEARL

A positive skin prick test occurs when antigen-specific IgE (bound to mast cells) crosslinks and causes histamine to be released.

Anaphylaxis

Etiology

- Foods
- Insects
- Latex
- Medications
- Idiopathic

Treatment

- Oxygen
- Subcutaneous **epinephrine** diluted to 1:1000 administered at 0.01 mg/kg (max: 0.3 ml). May be repeated at 15-minute intervals.
- Followed by
  - Antihistamines
  - Corticosteroids
  - Beta$_2$-agonist as needed
  - Intravenous fluids

Diagnosis

- Obtain **tryptase level** to confirm mast cell degranulation

Immunizations with History of Egg Allergy

MEASLES, MUMPS AND RUBELLA
- Does not contain significant egg cross-reacting protein
- **Do not need skin testing** prior to administration
- All children should receive immunization (even with history of egg anaphylaxis)

INFLUENZA
- Contains egg protein
- Children with history of anaphylaxis **should not** receive immunization
- Less severe reactions to eggs/feathers are not contraindications and do not warrant skin testing

YELLOW FEVER
- Contains egg protein
- **Skin testing** prior to administration is recommended in patients with history of systemic anaphylactic reactions
- Less severe reactions to eggs/feathers are not contraindications and do not warrant skin testing

Risk Factors for Latex Allergy

- **Spina bifida**
- Urologic abnormalities
- Health care worker
- Latex industry workers
- Food allergy—bananas, kiwi, avocados, cherries, plums, and chestnuts
- Repeated surgeries
- Unexplained intraoperative anaphylaxis

Drugs that Interfere with Allergy Skin Tests

- Anti-H_1 histamines (anti-H_2 histamines *do not* interfere with test)
- Imipramines (tricyclic antidepressants)
- Phenothiazines

Drug Reactions

FIXED DRUG ERUPTION
- Reaction occurs in **same place each time** drug is ingested
- New reaction can also occur with successive ingestions
- Typically round plaque, purple/red
- Associated with barbiturates, salicylates, phenacetin, phenolphthalein
- Treatment: avoidance of associated medications

TOXIC EPIDERMAL NECROLYSIS
- Hypersensitivity reaction to drug
- Associated with **sulfonamides**, amoxicillin, phenobarbitol and hydantoin
- Fever, skin pain, diffuse erythema and full-thickness skin loss
- **Nikolsky sign:** denudation of skin with gentle pressure
- Treated as "burn patient" in ICU

PHOTOTOXIC DRUG REACTION
- An exaggerated sunburn response to ultra-violet light
- **Burning sensation**, can be pruritic
- Associated with **sulfonamides**, NSAIDs, **doxycycline and tetracycline**
- Also can occur with skin contact of certain psoralen-containing foods, including lemons, limes, and celery

REFERENCES

1. Behrman R, Kliegman R, Jenson H: Nelson Textbook of Pediatrics, 17th edition, Philadelphia, W.B. Saunders, 2003.

2. Middleton E, Reed C, Ellis E, Adkinson N, Yunginger J, Busse W: Allergy Principles & Practice (Volumes I and II), 5th edition, St. Louis, Mosby, 1998.

3. AAP Red Book 2000, 25th edition, 2000.

4. Weinberg S, Prose N, Kristal L: Color Atlas of Pediatric Dermatology, 3rd edition, New York, McGraw-Hill, 1998.

5. Kane K, Ryder J, Johnson R, etal: Color Atlas and Synopsis of Pediatric Dermatology, New York, McGraw-Hill, 2002.

6. Executive Summary of the NAEPP Expert Panel Report: Guidelines for the Diagnosis and Management of Asthma—Update on Selected Topics 2002. NIH Publication, June 2002.

CARDIOLOGY

Diagnostic Evaluation of a Cyanotic Neonate

STEP 1:

Hyperoxia Test
- Blood gas done at room air
- Blood gas done with child breathing 100% oxygen

Interpretation
- If $PaO_2 > 200$ mmHg on 100% O_2—no congenital heart disease
- If $PaO_2 < 150$ mmHg on 100% O_2—suggests cardiac lesion with mixing (no restricted pulmonary blood flow)
- If $PaO_2 < 50$ mmHg on 100% O_2—parallel blood flow or a mixing lesion with restricted pulmonary blood flow

> **PEARL**
>
> Cannot use a pulse oximeter for hyperoxia test.

STEP 2:
Pulse oximetry at preductal (right hand) and postductal (left foot) sites

Interpretation
- If preductal saturation is greater than postductal saturation a "differential cyanosis" exists. It occurs with:
  - Persistent pulmonary hypertension of the newborn
  - Left ventricular outflow tract obstruction
    —Aortic stenosis
    —Aortic atresia
  - If postductal saturation is greater than preductal a "reverse differential"cyanosis exists.

> **PEARL**
>
> "Reverse differential" cyanosis only occurs in **transposition of the great arteries.**

STEP 3:
EKG

STEP 4:
Chest radiograph

Cyanotic Cardiac Lesions

CARDIAC LESION	EKG FINDINGS	CHEST X-RAY	CARDIAC EXAM
Truncus arteriosus	**Right and left ventricular hypertrophy**	Increased pulmonary markings Cardiomegaly	Holosystolic murmur Loud S_2
d-Transposition of the great arteries	Normal in newborn	Increased pulmonary markings **"Egg-shaped" heart**	**Single loud S_2** Usually no murmur
Total anomalous pulmonary venous return without obstruction (supracardiac 50%)	Right axis deviation Right ventricular hypertrophy	Increased pulmonary markings **"Snowman"-shaped heart**	Wide and fixed S_2
Tricuspid atresia	**Left axis deviation Left ventricular hypertrophy**	Decreased pulmonary markings Normal heart size	Holosystolic murmur
Tetralogy of Fallot	Right axis deviation Right ventricular hypertrophy	Decreased pulmonary markings **"Boot-shaped" heart**	Holosystolic murmur Right ventricular heave Systolic ejection murmur
Ebstein's anomaly	Right bundle branch block Wolf-Parkinson-White syndrome	Decreased pulmonary markings **Severe cardiomegaly**	Tricuspid regurgitation Fixed split S_2
Hypoplastic left heart syndrome	Normal	Increased pulmonary markings Cardiomegaly	Loud Single S_2

Noncyanotic Heart Lesions

CARDIAC LESION	EKG FINDINGS	CHEST X-RAY	CARDIAC EXAM
Atrial septal defect	Right ventricular hypertrophy	Increased pulmonary markings Cardiomegaly	**Fixed split S_2**
Ventricular septal defects (small)	Normal	Normal	Holosystolic murmur (loud)
Ventricular septal defects (large)	Left atrial and ventricular hypertrophy Right ventricular hypertrophy	Increased pulmonary markings Cardiomegaly	Holosystolic murmur Prominent S_2
Patent Ductus Arteriosus (Large)	Right and left ventricular hypertrophy	Increased pulmonary markings Cardiomegaly	**"Machinery murmur"** (continuous)
Aortic stenosis	Left ventricular hypertrophy ST depressions Inverted T waves	Normal or increased pulmonary markings Cardiomegaly	Harsh systolic ejection murmur at *right* upper sternal border Ejection **click**
Pulmonic stenosis	Right ventricular hypertrophy Right axis deviation	Normal or decreased pulmonary markings Normal heart size	Harsh systolic ejection murmur at *left* upper sternal border Ejection **click**

Arrhythmia Treatments

SUPRAVENTRICULAR TACHYCARDIA
- Vagal stimulation (ice bag on face)
- Adenosine
- Digoxin
- Synchronized DC cardioversion in unstable patients

WOLFF-PARKINSON-WHITE
- Short PR interval with slow upstroke of the QRS **(delta wave)**
- Radiofrequency ablation if symptomatic

ATRIAL FLUTTER
- **"Saw tooth" waves** on EKG
- Can be normal finding in neonate
- DC cardioversion
- Digoxin

ATRIAL FIBRILLATION
- Frequently seen due to rheumatic mitral valve disease
- Best initial treatment: digoxin

SINUS BRADYCARDIA
- Heart rate < 60 beats/min
- Frequently seen in athletes (athletes also have **large hearts**)
- No treatment necessary

VENTRICULAR TACHYCARDIA
- Intravenous lidocaine if stable
- Synchronized cardioversion if unstable

VENTRICULAR FIBRILLATION
- External cardiac massage
- DC defibrillation

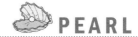

PEARL

Do not use **digoxin** because it may lead to atrial fibrillation and/or ventricular fibrillation.

Pericarditis

Etiology

COLLAGEN VASCULAR DISEASES
- Juvenile rheumatoid arthritis
- Systemic lupus erythematosus

INFECTIONS
- Viral (coxsackie, influenza)
- Bacterial
- Tuberculosis

SURGICAL COMPLICATION
- Post-pericardiotomy syndrome
  - 1 to 2 weeks after heart surgery

Manifestations
- Chest pain (worse in the *supine position*)
- Visible jugular pulsations
- Distant heart sounds
- Pulsus paradox

Exam Findings
- Cardiac rub

Chest X-Ray
- "Water bottle" heart

EKG Findings
- **Low voltages**
- **S-T elevations**
- Electrical alterans

Diagnosis
- Echocardiography

Management
- Small effusion—anti-inflammatory medications
- Large effusion—pericardiocentesis

Risks
- **Cardiac tamponade** (if not treated)

Hypertrophic Cardiomyopathy

Inheritance
- Autosomal dominant

Pathophysiology
- Septum becomes thickened with stiff left ventricle
- Abnormal diastolic function
- Normal systolic function

Manifestations
- Dyspnea with exertion
- Chest pain
- **Syncope**

Cardiac Findings
- Bisferious pulse (double-peaked)
- Ventricular gallop
- Murmurs (ejection or regurgitation)

EKG
- Left axis deviation
- Left ventricular hypertrophy
- Possible ST and T wave changes secondary to strain

Diagnosis
- Echocardiogram

Treatment
- Beta-blockers
- Calcium channel blockers

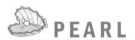 **P E A R L**

Standing and the Valsalva maneuver **increase** the intensity of the ejection murmur secondary to increasing the outflow obstruction.

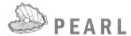 **P E A R L**

Must avoid competitive sports because exertion is a risk for sudden death.

Kawasaki Disease

Diagnosis

NEED FIVE OF SIX OF THE CRITERIA

- Fever ($>$ 40° C) for 5 days or longer
- Bilateral nonexudative conjunctivitis
- Cervical lymphadenopathy
- Fissured, dry and bright red swollen lips
- Erythema and swelling of hands/feet
- Maculopapular eruption on the trunk

Complications

- **Coronary artery aneurysms**
- Myopericarditis
- Thrombocytosis (650,000–2,000,000/mm^3)
- Hydrops of the gallbladder
- Sterile pyuria (urethritis)
- Aseptic meningitis
- Joint pain

Work-up

- Echocardiography at diagnosis, 6 to 8 weeks and 6 to 12 months

Treatment

- **IVIG**
- **Aspirin**
    - —High dose (100 mg/kg/24 hr) in acute phase
    - —Low dose (3–5 mg/kg/24 hr) until labs normal

Prognosis

- Untreated—25 % risk of coronary artery aneurysm

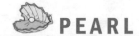

PEARL

Irritability is severe in children with Kawasaki disease.

Coarctation of the Aorta

Manifestations

INFANT WITH CRITICAL STENOSIS
- Murmur—systolic ejection murmur heard at apex
- Shock
- Congestive heart failure
  - Sweating with feeds
  - Feed slowly
  - Wheezing
  - Failure to thrive

CHILD WITH MILD STENOSIS
- **Asymptomatic hypertension** on well child exam

EKG Findings

Neonate: right ventricular hypertrophy
Child: left ventricular hypertrophy

Radiographic Finding

CHEST RADIOGRAPH
- Classic finding: **rib notching** (takes years to develop)
- "3" sign secondary to dilated descending aorta

BARIUM SWALLOW
- Dilated descending aorta forms an "E"

Diagnosis

WORK-UP:
- Initially, check **four extremity pulses and blood pressure**
- Echocardiography

Treatment
- Surgical

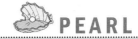

PEARL

Must consider Turner syndrome in a female with coarctation of the aorta.

Rheumatic Heart Disease

Etiology

- **Untreated** group A beta-hemolytic *Streptococcus* infection
- Pharyngeal infections but *not skin infections*

Jones' Criteria

MAJOR
- Migratory polyarthritis (knees/elbows/ankles and wrists)
- Carditis
- Subcutaneous nodules
- Erythema marginatum
- Chorea

MINOR
- Fever
- Prolonged PR
- Increased ESR
- Arthralgia

Diagnosis

- Two majors *or*
  One major and two minor *with*
    evidence of a recent streptococcal infection

Cardiac Manifestations

- **Mitral regurgitation** (most common)
- Mitral stenosis
- Aortic stenosis
- Aortic regurgitation

Treatment

- Penicillin
- Aspirin
- Prednisone

Prophylaxis

- IM penicillin G benzathine every 28 days in all cases
- Use erythromycin for patients allergic to penicillin

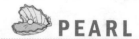

PEARL

Symptoms begin **2 to 6 weeks after pharyngitis.**

Hypertension

Criteria
- Elevated blood pressure above the 95th percentile for age
- Persistent: occurring on **three** separate occasions
- Standardized measurement techniques used

Differential Diagnosis
- Cardiac disease (coarctation of aorta)
- **Renal disease**
- History of umbilical artery catheterization
- Renal artery stenosis (exam with **abdominal bruit**)
- Essential hypertension
- Endocrine disorders
- Neurologic disorders

Initial Work-up
LABORATORY STUDIES
- BUN/Cr
- CBC
- Electrolytes
- Urine analysis/culture

PROCEDURES
- Renal ultrasound
- Chest radiograph

Treatment
FIRST LINE
- Diet control (low salt)
- Weight loss
- Exercise

SECOND LINE
- Diuretics
- Beta-blockers
- ACE inhibitors
- Calcium channel blockers

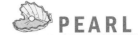

PEARL

Air bladder in cuff should be wide enough to cover 75% of the upper limb. If cuff is too small, it causes a falsely *elevated* blood pressure.

Long QT Syndrome

Inheritance
- Variable; many are familial

Syndromes with Long QT
ROMANO-WARD SYNDROME
- Autosomal dominant

JERVELL AND LANGE-NIELSEN SYNDROME
- Autosomal recessive
- Can be associated with **deafness**

Definition
- QTc > .46, where QTc = QT / square root of RR

Presentations
- Syncope, seizures and sudden death

Treatment
- Beta-blockers
- Pacemakers

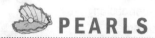 **PEARLS**

Cases of near sudden death have been reported with loud alarms and hitting the water during a dive secondary to a sudden catecholamine surge.

Sudden death or near sudden death *precipitated by exercise* should be ruled out for anomalous/aberrant coronary artery.

Postural Orthostatic Tachycardia Syndrome (POTS)

Definition
- Episodic sinus tachycardia and chest discomfort
- Intolerance to prolonged upright positioning occurs

Family History
- History of syncope or "fainting"

Orthostatic Testing
- Normal blood pressure and pulse

Tilt Table Testing
- Abnormal—tachycardia, chest tightness, light-headedness

Exam
- Normal

30-Day Event Recorder
- Normal

REFERENCES

1. Behrman R, Kliegman R, Jenson H: Nelson Textbook of Pediatrics, 17th edition, Philadelphia, W.B. Saunders, 2003.

2. Park M: Pediatric Cardiology for Practitioners, 4th edition, St. Louis, Mosby, 2002.

3. Braunwald E: Heart Disease—A Textbook of Cardiovascular Medicine, 6th edition, Philadelphia, W.B. Saunders, 2001.

DERMATOLOGY

Malignant Melanoma

Signs
- Asymmetry or irregularity in shape
- Border changes: projections/invaginations
- Color changes—darkening/lightening; new reds, blacks, blues, or browns
- Diameter greater than 6 mm

Diagnosis
- Biopsy

Prevention
- Sun protection factor (SPF) $\geq$ 15 (against UVA and UVB)

Prognosis
- Related to thickness/depth of penetration
- Poor for deep/metastatic lesions

Acne Management

COMEDONAL ACNE ("BLACKHEADS" AND "WHITEHEADS")

Management
- Topical retinoids, benzoyl peroxide, antibiotics and desquamating agents (salicylic acid)

INFLAMMATORY ACNE

Management
FIRST LINE
- Topical retinoids, benzoyl peroxide, antibiotics and desquamating agents (salicylic acid)

SECOND LINE
- Oral antibiotics (tetracycline)

NODULOCYSTIC ACNE

Management
FIRST LINE
- Topical retinoids, benzoyl peroxide, antibiotics, desquamating agents (salicylic acid)

SECOND LINE
- Oral antibiotics

THIRD LINE
- **Oral isotretinoin**

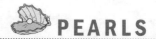

PEARLS

Isotretinoin is reserved for patients who fail treatment. Adolescent females must be using an **effective form of contraception** before isotretinoin is started because it is a potent teratogen.

Androgens are associated with acne (and axillary hair) in males and females.

Psoriasis

Rash

- Erythematous papules
- **Symmetric silver/yellow-white plaques** (sharp borders)
- Nonpruritic

Location

- Knees
- Elbows
- Genital area
- Scalp
- Intergluteal fold

Manifestations

- **Koebner phenomenon** (rash occurs at site of trauma)
- Onycholysis (separation of the nail plate from nail bed)
- **Auspitz sign** (capillary bleeding when scale pulled off)
- **Pitted nails**

Complications

- Arthritis

Treatment

- Skin hydration
- Tar
- Sunlight/ultraviolet B light
- Corticosteroids

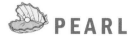

PEARL

Guttate psoriasis occurs following streptococcal infections and manifests as an explosive onset of small oval/round lesions on the trunk, face and limbs.

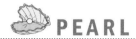

PEARL

Koebner phenomenon is a valuable diagnostic tool.

Ichthyosis

ICHTHYOSIS VULGARIS

Inheritance

- Autosomal dominant

Manifestations

- Atopy/keratosis pilaris
- Occurs in first year of life
- Scaling (**"pasted-on" appearance**)
- Usually on extensor surfaces of extremities (**shins**)

Treatment

- Baths with bath oil
- Keratolytics such as lactic acid, urea and glycolic acids
- Emollients—prevent evaporation
- Salicylic acid—control scaling

LAMELLAR ICHTHYOSIS

Inheritance

- Autosomal recessive

Manifestations

- Evident at birth; newborns have a **collodion membrane**
- Membrane is shed and large **plate-like scales** form
- Scales involve the *entire body* (including face)
- Pruritic

Treatment

- Prolonged baths with bath oil
- Emollients—prevent evaporation
- Keratolytic agents: lactic acid, urea and glycolic acids

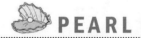

PEARL

Do not restrict bathing under the assumption that it will dry the skin. Hydration (bathing) helps minimize the symptoms/malodor.

Pityriasis Rosea

Epidemiology

- Typically occurs with 4- to 20-year olds in winter/spring

Rash

- Starts with 2- to 5-cm annular scaly patch **(herald patch)**
- Followed by symmetric, scaly, oval, pink/red lesions
- Lesions covered with fine scale **(crinkly appearance)**
- Follows the lines of skin cleavage:
    - —Back (**"Christmas tree"** pattern)
    - —Limbs
    - —Hands, face and feet

Diagnosis

- Clinical

Treatment

- Usually self-limited over 2 to 3 months

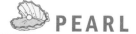

PEARL

Herald patch can be mistaken for tinea corporis.

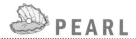

PEARL

Syphilis must be ruled out in any sexually active patient with this rash due to its resemblance to secondary syphilis.

Foot Dermatitis

DYSHIDROTIC ECZEMA
- **Symmetric** involvement of **bottom of feet** (soles and palms)
- Papules/vesicles (acute phase) and lichenification (chronic phase)
- Intensely pruritic
- Pathogenesis: unknown
- Associated with hyperhidrosis
- Treatment: topical steroids and lubricants

ALLERGIC CONTACT DERMATITIS
- T-cell mediated hypersensitivity
- **Symmetric** involvement of **top of feet**
- Usually from leather of chemicals in shoes/shoe rubber
- Pruritic
- Treatment: elimination of contact with allergen; topical steroids

TINEA PEDIS
- **Asymmetric**
- Involves **toe webs** (third to fourth, fourth to fifth) and **bottom of feet**
- Subtle scaling involving the fourth toe web space is classic during symptom-free periods
- Fungal mycelia seen with KOH preparation
- Pruritic with foul odor
- Treatment: Topical antifungals; keep feet dry

Stevens-Johnson Syndrome

Etiology

- Infectious (i.e., *Mycoplasma pneumoniae* and *Herpes*)
- Drugs (sulfonamides, NSAIDS and anticonvulsants)

Manifestations

CUTANEOUS FEATURES
- Erythematous macules
- Macules develop into vesicles, bullae, and ulcers
- Hemorrhagic crusting
- Occurs on face, trunk and extremities
- **Painful**
- Must involve two or more mucosal surfaces:
  - Eyes
  - Oral cavity
  - Esophagus/GI
  - Anogenital

Complications

- Bacterial superinfection
- Eye (corneal ulcers, uveitis)
- Myocarditis
- Renal failure secondary to acute tubular necrosis
- Hepatitis

Treatment

- Supportive/symptomatic (treated similar to burn patients)

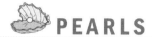 **PEARLS**

Ophthalmology must be consulted to monitor for ocular sequelae.

No double-blind studies have shown that corticosteroids are advocated for treatment; actually steroids may increase risk of sepsis.

Alopecia

TRICHOTILLOMANIA
- Hair loss secondary to repetitive twirling, plucking or rubbing
- Results from habit, stress or obsessive-compulsive disorder
- Exam: **irregular patch of hair loss with hairs of different lengths**

TELOGEN EFFLUVIUM
- Hair loss secondary to a significant stress (childbirth, serious infection)
- Hair falls out 2 to 4 months after stressful event
- Etiology: hair follicles convert to resting state
- Exam: **diffuse alopecia** without erythema or scaling

TINEA CAPITIS
- Hair loss secondary to infection with *T. tonsurans* or *M. canis*
- Exam: **"black dot", broken hairs with erythema and scaling**
- Diagnosis: KOH preparation or fungal culture
- Treatment is with griseofulvin and selenium shampoo

ALOPECIA AREATA
- Hair loss secondary to immune dysregulation
- Exam: **localized patchy hair loss;** no redness, scaling or broken hairs
- Patients can lose eyebrows, eyelashes (**"alopecia totalis"**)
- Patients can lose all body hair (**"alopecia universalis"**)
- Prognosis: 95% of children regrow hair in 1 year without treatment

Miscellaneous Rashes

IMPETIGO
- Nonbullous impetigo
  - Papules form vesicles then pustules
  - **"Honey-like" exudates**
  - *S. aureus* and Group A beta-hemolytic streptococcus
- Bullous impetigo
  - Macules form bullae (can be several centimeters)
  - "Varnish-like"coating forms over denuded areas
  - *S. aureus*
- Treatment: PO dicloxacillin or cephalexin

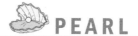

PEARL

Treatment of impetigo **does not** prevent the development of post-streptococcal glomeru-lonephritis.

PAPULAR URTICARIA
- Occurs in toddlers
- Pruritic papules
- Pathogenesis: **delayed hypersensitivity to insect bites**
- Treatment: avoidance and antihistamines

ERYTHEMA TOXICUM NEONATORUM
- Occurs in newborn infants
- Onset occurs during **first 3 days of life**
- Occurs anywhere but usually spares perioral, palms and soles
- Lesions are erythematous macules, vesicles and pustules
- **Gram stain: eosinophils**
- Treatment: none needed

NEONATAL PUSTULAR MELANOSIS
- Occurs more commonly in newborn black infants
- Always present at birth or **first 24 hours of life**
- Occurs on face, hands, feet typically
- Pustules rupture leaving hyperpigmented macules
- **Gram stain: neutrophils**
- Treatment: none needed

Molluscum Contagiosum

Etiology

- Pox virus

Incubation

- 2 to 7 weeks

Manifestations

- Translucent or **white ("pearly") papules**
- Central dimple or umbilication
- Occur mainly on the face, neck, axillae and thighs

Treatment

- Resolves spontaneously
- Curettage/freezing if cosmetically warranted

Head Lice

Etiology

- *Pediculus humanus capitis*

Manifestations

- Common in school-aged children
- Transmitted by direct contact/indirect contact (hats/combs)
- Intensely pruritic

Diagnosis

- Nits, nymphs and lice can be seen by naked eye

Treatment

- 1% permethrin cream (repeat in 1 week)—first choice
- Lindane
- Wash linens
- Brushes/combs cleaned or discarded
- Must treat all family members

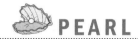 **PEARL**

Lindane causes neurotoxicity; avoid in infants, young children and pregnant/breast-feeding women.

Dermatologic Pearls

HEMANGIOMAS
- Can expand for first 2 years of life and then will involute
- **Kasabach-Merritt phenomenon** (hemolytic anemia, thrombocytopenia and coagulopathy) occurs in rapidly enlarging lesion
- Can be associated with airway obstruction
- Treatment: pulse-dye laser

PYOGENIC GRANULOMA
- Benign vascular tumor
- 2- to 10-mm pedunculated papule
- **Very friable; bleeds profusely**
- Treatment: cauterization (bleeding) and pulse-dye laser

ACANTHOSIS NIGRICANS
- **Grey-brown velvety plaques** on axillae, neck and groin
- Associated with Type II diabetes mellitus in obese children
- May herald polycystic ovarian disease

TINEA VERSICOLOR
- Etiology: *P. orbiculare or M. furfur*
- Occurs in adolescents and young adults
- Rash typically involves back, chest, neck and upper arms
- Lesions are hypo/hyperpigmented with fine scale
- KOH preparation: "spaghetti and meatballs" appearance
- Wood lamp: yellow or gold fluorescence
- Treatment: selenium shampoo, topical or oral antifungals

REFERENCES

1. Behrman R, Kliegman R, Jenson H: Nelson Textbook of Pediatrics, 17th edition, Philadelphia, W.B. Saunders 2003.

2. Kane K, Ryder J, Johnson R, etal: Color Atlas and Synopsis of Pediatric Dermatology, New York, McGraw-Hill, 2002.

3. Weston W, Lane A, Morelli J: Color Textbook of Pediatric Dermatology, 3rd edition, St. Louis, Mosby, 2002.

4. AAP Red Book 2000, 25th edition, 2000.

5. Weinberg S, Prose N, Kristal L. Color Atlas of Pediatric Dermatology, 3rd edition, New York, McGraw-Hill, 1998.

DEVELOPMENT

CHAPTER

5

Sexual Maturity Rating (SMR)

MALES

SMR 1: Prepubertal
SMR 2: Testes increase in size and volume
Scrotum becomes reddened, thinner and textured
Long, downy hair
SMR 3: Penis increases in length
Testes increase in size
Pubic hair changes to coarse, curly and pigmented
SMR 4: Penis length and circumference increase
Pubic hair becomes more curly and dense
SMR 5: Male phallus and scrotum are adult size
Pubic hair extends to thighs

FEMALES

SMR 1: Prepubertal
SMR 2: Small breast buds
Long, downy pubic hair
SMR 3: Breast tissue extends beyond areolar perimeter
Pubic hair changes to coarse, curly and pigmented
SMR 4: Breasts enlarge
Secondary mound forms from the areola and papilla
Pubic hair becomes more curly and dense
SMR 5: Breast at adult size
No longer a separate mound of areola from breast
Pubic hair extends to thighs

Puberty

FEMALES

Age
■ Between 8 and 13 years old

First Sign
■ Breast bud formation (average 11.2 years)

Duration
■ Completed in approximately 4 years (1.5- to 8-year range)

Growth Spurt
■ Usually begins 1 year *before* breast development

Peak Height Velocity
■ Occurs at SMR 3 and 4 (approximately 9 cm/yr)

Menarche
■ Average age: 12.8 years
■ Range 10 to 16 years
■ Usually occurs 2 to 2.5 years after breast development begins
■ Usually occurs 3.3 years after the growth spurt

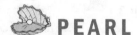

When menstruation occurs:
—10% by SMR 2
—30% by SMR 3
—90% by SMR 4
—100% by SMR 5

MALES

Age
■ Occurs between 9 and 14 years old

First Sign
■ Testicular enlargement (11.5 years)

Peak Height Velocity
■ SMR of 3 and 4 (approximately 10 cm/yr)

Duration
■ Completed in 3.5 years (2- to 5-year range)

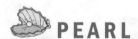

Gynecomastia can normally occur during puberty in males.

Speech Development

3 months
- Coos

6 months
- Babbles

8 months
- "Dada/mama" indiscriminately

10 months
- "Dada/mama" discriminately

12 Months
- One to three words
- Rarely understood

24 Months
- Two to three word phrases
- Understood 50% of time by strangers

36 Months
- Sentences
- Understood 85% of time by strangers

48 Months
- Understood 100% of time by strangers

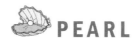 **PEARL**

Any delay of speech development should be initially investigated with a hearing evaluation.

Motor Milestones

3 months

- Holds head up steadily
- Hands held open at rest

6 months

- Transfer an object from hand to hand
- Sit in arm-propped position
- Raking grasp
- Roll over in both directions

12 months

- Pincer grasp (pick up a raisin)
- Few independent steps
- Drink from a cup with assistance
- Follow simple commands with a gesture

18 months

- Build a tower of four blocks
- Release a raisin into a bottle
- Spontaneous scribbling
- Walk backwards

24 months

- Throw ball overhand
- Build a tower of six or more blocks
- Wash/dry hands
- Remove clothing
- Jump with two feet off the floor
- Copy a vertical line

Motor Milestones *continued*

36 months

- Copy a circle
- Pedals a tricycle
- Uses alternate feet walking up steps
- Dries hands
- Dresses/undresses partially

48 months

- Copy a cross
- Hops/skips
- Uses alternate feet walking down steps

5 year olds

- Copy a square
- Skips alternating feet
- Jumps over low obstacles
- Ties shoes

6 year olds

- Copy a diamond/triangle

Response to Stress

PARENTAL DIVORCE

Preschool Child
- Regression

Early School-Age Child
- Open grieving, including sobbing

Late School-Age Child
- Anger

Adolescents
- Depression/suicidal ideation

DEATH OF CLOSE FAMILY MEMBER

Preschool Child
- Regression, temper tantrums or anger

School-Age Child
- Somatic complaints (headaches, stomach aches)
- Sleep disturbances
- Deterioration of school performance

Adolescents
- Depression/suicidal ideation

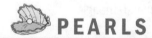

PEARLS

Kubler-Ross Stages of Grief
- —Denial
- —Anger
- —Bargaining
- —Depression
- —Acceptance

REFERENCES

1. Zitelli B, Davis H: Atlas of Pediatric Physical Diagnosis, 4th edition, St. Louis, Mosby, 2002.

2. Behrman R, Kliegman R, Jenson H: Nelson Textbook of Pediatrics, 17th edition, Philadelphia, W.B. Saunders, 2003.

3. McMillan J, DeAngelis C, Feigin R, Warshaw J: Oski's Pediatrics—Principles and Practice, 3rd edition, Philadelphia, Lippincott, Williams & Wilkins, 1999.

4. Rudolph C, Rudolph A, Hostetter M, Lister G, Siegel N: Rudolph's Pediatrics, 21st edition, New York, McGraw–Hill, 2002.

5. Siberry G, Iannone R: The Harriet Lane Handbook, 15th edition, St. Louis, Mosby, 2000.

Ear, Nose and Throat

Otitis Media with Effusion (OME)

Definition
- Fluid in inner ear without signs/symptoms of inflammation

Etiology

ABNORMAL EUSTACHIAN TUBE FUNCTION
- Increased tube compliance or inactive opening mechanism

MECHANICAL OBSTRUCTION
- Intrinsic: inflammation (allergens, infections or smoke)
- Extrinsic: adenoid hypertrophy

Manifestations
- Conductive hearing loss
- Delayed speech and language development

Treatment
- Less than 3 months of OME observation
- 3 months of OME beta-lactamase–resistant antibiotic in untreated patients
- More than 4 to 6 months of OME bilateral myringotomy tubes

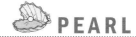 **PEARL**

Studies have shown that decongestants and anti-histamines are ineffective for treatment, whereas efficacy of intranasal steroids/systemic steroids is unproven.

Chronic Suppurative Otitis Media

Manifestations

- Chronic inflammation of the middle ear
- Otorrhea
- Nonintact tympanic membrane (perforation/BMT)
- Refractory to medical treatment for > 6 weeks

Etiology

- *P. aeruginosa*
- *S. aureus*
- Anaerobes (i.e., *Bacteroides, Peptostreptococcus*)

Management

- PO antibiotics; if refractory, use IV antibiotics

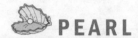

PEARL

Associated with **cholesteatoma**.

Acute Otitis Media

Etiology

- Viral
- Bacterial
    - *S. pneumoniae* (30–50%)
    - nontypeable H. *influenzae* (20–30%)
    - M. *catarrhalis* (1–5%)

Risk for Resistant S. pneumoniae

- Recent antibiotics (prior month)
- < 2 years of age
- Daycare

Treatment Options

Low Risk for resistant S. pneumoniae

- High-dose (80 mg/kg/day) amoxicillin *or*
- Low dose (45 mg/kg/day) amoxicillin

High Risk for resistant S. pneumoniae

- High-dose (80 mg/kg/day) amoxicillin or
- High-dose amoxicillin-clavulanate (80 mg/kg/day) or
- Cefuroxime (30 mg/kg/day)

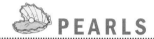 **PEARLS**

Treatment failure (after 3 days) is defined as lack of clinical improvement (pain/fever), otorrhea or a bulging tympanic membrane. Treatment failures require an alternative treatment.

Cholesteatoma

Definition
- Accumulation of keratinizing squamous epithelium
- Occurs within the middle ear and mastoid cavity

Manifestations
- **White, shiny, greasy debris**
- **Foul-smelling** discharge
- Erosion of the ossicles, inner ear/temporal bone

Treatment
- Surgery

Indications for Tonsillectomy and Adenoidectomy

TONSILLECTOMY AND ADENOIDECTOMY
- Obstructive sleep apnea
- Hypertrophic tonsils/adenoids

TONSILLECTOMY
- Recurrent group A beta-hemolytic streptococcal infections
  - Seven infections in 1 year
  - Five infections/year for 2 consecutive years
  - More than three infections/year for 3 consecutive years

ADENOIDECTOMY
- Repeated otitis media infection (acute and OME)
- Chronic mouth breathing/hyponasal speech

Otitis Externa ("Swimmer's Ear")

Definition

- Inflammation of the external ear canal

Manifestations

- Redness
- Swelling
- Tenderness of the auricle and/or the ear canal

Risks for Infection

- Swimming
- Trauma (i.e., use of Q-tips)

Treatment

- Analgesics
- Antimicrobial-corticosteroid ototopical solutions

Prevention

- **Isopropyl alcohol/acetic acid solution** after swimming

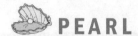 **PEARL**

Malignant otitis externa (cellulitis/vasculitis due to *S. aureus* and *P. aeruginosa* that extends into the deep surrounding tissues of the neck) requires IV antibiotics. Occurs with immunocompromised patients and patients with diabetes mellitus.

Etiology of Hoarse Voice

Congenital
- Vocal cord paralysis
- Laryngeal webs, cysts or clefts
- Subglottic stenosis

Trauma
- Intubation injury (unilateral/bilateral vocal cord paralysis)

Inflammatory
- Infection
- Allergy
- GERD
- Angioneurotic edema of larynx

Physiologic
- Nodules

Neoplastic
- Papilloma (history of genital warts with mother)

Endocrine
- Hypothyroidism
- Hypocalcemia

Rheumatologic
- Juvenile rheumatoid arthritis

Iatrogenic
- Recurrent laryngeal nerve injury from surgery

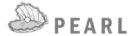 **PEARL**

Common cause of chronic *acquired* hoarseness usually secondary to overuse of voice "screamers nodules".

Neck Masses

DIAGNOSIS	LOCATION	DIAGNOSTIC COMMENTS
Thyroglossal duct cyst	Midline	**Moves up/down with swallowing** Retracts with tongue protrusion
Branchial cysts	Anterior triangle	Rarely evident until later in life Associated with fistulas
Cystic hygroma	Posterior triangle	**Soft/spongy** with palpation
Teratoma	Midline	**Calcifications**
Dermoid cysts	Midline	Doughy
Hemangioma	Variable	Increase with Valsalva maneuver
Congenital torticollis	Lateral	**Solid mass in sternocleidomastoid**
Cervical adenitis	Variable	*B. henselae* (cat-scratch disease) Nontuberculous mycobacteria Viral Bacterial *(S. aureus)*

Stridor

INSPIRATORY STRIDOR (SUPRAGLOTTIC LESION)

- Laryngomalacia (most common)
  - Classically presents at birth
  - **Worse in supine position**
  - Nasopharyngoscopy reveals a rolled, omega-shaped epiglottis
  - Usually resolves by 18 months
- Infection (croup, tracheitis, retropharyngeal abscess, epiglottitis)
- Tumor
- Bilateral vocal cord paralysis
  - Diagnosed with nasopharyngoscopy or airway fluoroscopy
  - Associated with a **weak cry**

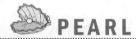 **PEARL**

Acquired subglottic stenosis is associated with prolonged intubation and usually presents 1 to 2 months after extubation.

BIPHASIC STRIDOR (GLOTTIC OR SUBGLOTTIC LESION)

- Hemangioma (associated with **cutaneous hemangioma**)
  - Microlaryngoscopy used to diagnose
- Subglottic stenosis (congenital or acquired)

EXPIRATORY STRIDOR (USUALLY INTRATHORACIC)

- Tracheomalacia (common)
  - Airway fluoroscopy and rigid/flexible bronchoscopy used to diagnose
- Bilateral vocal cord paralysis
- Foreign body (**watch for foreign body on chest film—board favorite!**)
- Tumor
- Vascular compression (i.e., subclavian vein, aberrant innominate artery)
  - Diagnosed with barium swallow with *posterior* esophageal indentation in vascular rings or subclavian artery/vein

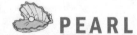 **PEARL**

Barium swallow will *not* identify anterior compression by innominate artery.

Choanal Atresia

UNILATERAL CHOANAL ATRESIA
- Usually *do not* present with respiratory distress
- Present later in life with **unilateral rhinorrhea** refractory to medications

BILATERAL CHOANAL ATRESIA
- Present in newborn period with respiratory distress with feeding and when mouth closed
- Diagnose by failure to pass a no. 6 French catheter through the nose
- Treated with surgical intervention
- Associated with CHARGE syndrome
  - **C**oloboma
  - **H**eart defects
  - **A**tresia choanal
  - **R**etarded growth/CNS development
  - **G**enitourinary anomalies
  - **E**ar anomalies/hearing loss

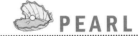

PEARL

Crying **relieves** respiratory distress (cyanosis) associated with bilateral choanal atresia.

REFERENCES

1. Pomeranz A, Busey S, Sabnis S: Pediatric Decision-Making Strategies, 1st edition, Philadelphia, W.B. Saunders, 2001.

2. Behrman R, Kliegman R, Jenson H: Nelson Textbook of Pediatrics, 17th edition, Philadelphia, W.B. Saunders, 2003.

3. McMillan J, DeAngelis C, Feigin R, Warshaw J: Oski's Pediatrics—Principles and Practice, 3rd edition, Philadelphia, Lippincott, Williams & Wilkins, 1999.

4. Rudolph C, Rudolph A, Hostetter M, Lister G, Siegel N: Rudolph's Pediatrics, 21st edition, New York, McGraw–Hill, 2002.

5. Bluestone C, Stool S, Kenna M: Pediatric Otolaryngology, 3rd edition, Philadelphia, W.B. Saunders, 1999.

Emergency Medicine/ Critical Care

Carbon Monoxide Poisoning

Sources
- Automobile engines ("long car rides")
- Fossil fuel burning
- House fire smoke

Prevalence
- Most common type of poisoning death

Manifestations
- Fatigue
- Headache
- Dizziness
- Nausea
- Confusion

Diagnosis
- COHgB level
- Oxygen saturation via co-oximetry

Treatment
- Removal of victim from CO source
- Oxygen by tight-fitting face mask
- Hyperbaric chamber for patients with:
    - COHgB > 25%
    - myocardial ischemia
    - neurologic symptoms
    - pregnant

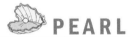

PEARL

"**Cherry-red gums**" may occur with poisoning.

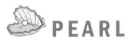

PEARL

Arterial PO_2 is normal (as is $HgBO_2$ *calculated* from PO_2), and pulse oximeter will give a **falsely high** reading. Must use co-oximetry.

Spider Bites

BROWN RECLUSE SPIDER (*LOXOSCELES RECLUSA*)

Description

- Small spider with *brown violin-shape* on cephalothorax

Manifestations

- Initially: minimal skin irritation
- Central blister develops with a whitish ring (target appearance)
- Over 3 to 4 days, local necrosis occurs with eventual ulceration
- Systemic symptoms:
    - Fever/chills
    - Vomiting
    - Joint pain
    - Petechial rash
    - Intravascular hemolysis
    - Hematuria/renal failure

Treatment

- Supportive

BLACK WIDOW (*LATRODECTUS MACTAM*)

Description

- Shiny black spider with *red hourglass shape* on ventral abdomen

Manifestations

- Bite site often unnoticed
- **Severe pain** at bite (within 12 hours)
- **Hypertension**
- **Painful cramping** of abdomen, lower back, chest and extremities
- Respiratory distress
- Priapism
- Seizures

Treatment

- Local wound care
- Narcotics/benzodiazepines
- Antihypertensives
- Antivenom is administered for:
    - Children < 40 kg
    - Respiratory distress
    - Seizures
    - Uncontrolled hypertension

Resuscitation Pearls

- Always remember ABCs: **Airway, Breathing** and **Circulation.**
- On the exam there will be many descriptions of scenarios in which the patient is obtunded, has altered mental status or is listless; **always establish an airway first.**
- Seizures should be managed with **IV lorazepam.**

Emergency Room Odors

ODOR	SOURCE	DISEASE
Sweet/fruity	Breath	Diabetic ketoacidosis
Musty/mousy	Body/urine	Phenylketonuria
Maple syrup	Urine	Maple syrup disease
Sweaty feet	Breath/body	Isovaleric academia
Almonds	Breath/body	Cyanide poisoning
Garlic	Body	Arsenic poisoning
Fishy/ammonia	Breath	Uremia
Fresh baked bread	Body	Typhoid fever
Pears	Body	Paraldehyde

Trauma

BLUNT ABDOMINAL TRAUMA
- CT scan is best initial radiologic study to assess injury

BLUNT GENITOURINARY TRAUMA
- Urethral injury (i.e., **blood at tip of penis**) must be ruled out via retrograde urethrography

TENSION PNEUMOTHORAX
- Trachea and mediastinum displace to opposite side of chest, impeding venous return and leading to respiratory distress, hypotension, and tachycardia
- Treatment is needle into the second intercostal space to decompress lung. *Do not* obtain chest x-ray first.

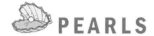

PEARLS

The most common organ injured in blunt abdominal trauma is the spleen (complain of left shoulder pain), followed by the liver and kidneys.

Duodenal and pancreatic injuries occur with bicycle handle bar injuries (child falls off bike and handle bars hit abdomen).

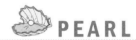

PEARL

Question will mention **tracheal deviation**, absent breath sounds, or tympanitic chest with percussion in cases of tension pneumothorax.

Head Trauma

BLUNT HEAD TRAUMA
- Initially perform CT scan of head to rule out fractures and bleeding

SUBDURAL HEMATOMA
- CT scan demonstrates **crescentric appearance**
- Usually bilateral
- Due to torn artery or bridging vein
- May develop over days to weeks after trauma
- Associated with severe acceleration/deceleration injuries
  - Shaken baby syndrome
  - Motor vehicle crashes

EPIDURAL HEMATOMA
- Usually with parietal bone fracture with laceration of middle meningeal artery
- CT demonstrates **biconcave appearance**
- Usually develops hours after injury
- Classic presentation: brief loss of consciousness, followed by lucid interval before deteriorating

BASILAR SKULL FRACTURE
- Associated with CSF rhinorrhea or otorrhea
- **Raccoon eyes**—periorbital ecchymosis
- **Battle's sign**—bruising over mastoids
- Blood behind tympanic membrane/hearing loss
- Clinically diagnosed secondary to *no radiologic evidence* in many cases

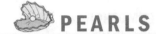 PEARLS

Ipsilateral dilated/unresponsive pupil, central hypoventilation and contralateral hemiparesis indicate an **uncal herniation** (compression of cranial nerve III).

Cushing triad (bradycardia, hypertension, and irregular respirations) is associated with severe increased intracranial pressure.

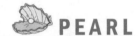 PEARL

CSF rhinorrhea will have **glucose in nasal discharge**.

Burns

Definitions

FIRST-DEGREE BURNS
- Epidermis only
- Red *without* blistering

SECOND-DEGREE BURNS
- Involve all epidermis and some dermis
- "Partial thickness burns"
- Red *with* blisters

THIRD-DEGREE BURNS
- All of epidermis/dermis
- "Full thickness burns"
- Gray/white
- Typically not painful

Treatment
- Cool water immediately
- Cleansing
- Silver sulfadiazine
- Dressing changes (BID) until reepithelialization

Recommended Hospitalization
- Second-degree burns > 5% of total body
- Third-degree burns > 1% of total body
- Circumferential burns
- Burns to hands, feet, genitalia, face or overlying joints
- Electrical burns
- Inhalation injury
- Chemical burns

Complications
- **Severe fluid losses**
- Infections

Ingestion Pearls

SYRUP OF IPECAC CONTRAINDICATIONS
- Signs of central nervous system depression
- Caustic ingestion
- Petroleum distillate ingestion
- Potential nervous system depressant ingestion
- More than 1 hour has elapsed between ingestion and presentation

GASTRIC LAVAGE
- Must be initiated within **1 hour of ingestion** or longer if toxin is known to slow gastric motility

SUBSTANCES POORLY ABSORBED BY CHARCOAL
- Iron
- Alcohol
- Cyanide
- Most hydrocarbons
- Most solvents

Ingestions

ASPIRIN

Sources
- Aspirin
- Salicylate-containing medications (oil of wintergreen)

Manifestation
- Increased respiratory rate/depth
- Fever
- Tachycardia
- Hypoglycemia
- **Hypokalemia**
- Liver toxicity
- Prolonged bleeding time
- Tinnitus

Treatment
- Charcoal
- Bicarbonate/potassium
- **Alkalinization** of urine
- IV fluids/electrolyte management
- Dialysis for renal, cardiac or hepatic failure

ORGANOPHOSPHATES

Source
- Pesticides (used in **rural/farming areas**)
- Can be absorbed via skin contact, inhalation or ingestion

Manifestation
- Constricted pupils
- **Profuse sweating/tearing/salivation**
- Abdominal cramping
- Wheezing/respiratory distress
- Nausea/vomiting

Treatment
- Wash skin immediately
- Activated charcoal for oral ingestion
- **Atropine and 2-pralidoxime**

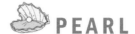

PEARL

A "wintergreen" breath odor may be mentioned in the description of the patient.

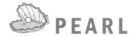

PEARL

Patients have both a respiratory alkalosis and metabolic acidosis.

Ingestions *continued*

TRICYCLIC ANTIDEPRESSANTS

Manifestations

- Hypertension/hypotension
- Tachycardia
- No consistent pupil findings
- Variable CNS effects:
    - —Coma
    - —Seizures
    - —Drowsiness

Treatment

- **Bicarbonate**
- Emesis is contraindicated

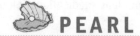

PEARL

Must monitor EKG for arrhythmias— prolonged QT and widened QRS.

OPIATES

Manifestations

- **Constricted pupils**
- **Decreased drive to breath**
- Depressed mental status

Treatment

- **Nalaxone**

BENZODIAZEPINE

Manifestations

- Normal pupils
- Mild decreased drive to breath
- Depressed mental status

Treatment

- **Flumazenil**

Ingestions *continued*

CORROSIVES

Manifestations
- Refusal to drink
- Salivation

Burns

ALKALINES (DRAIN CLEANERS)
- Produce liquefaction necrosis and can result in full-thickness injury and perforation of the esophagus/stomach

ACIDS (TOILET BOWL CLEANERS)
- Produce coagulation necrosis and eschar formation, which prevent full-thickness penetration

Management
- Oral administration of large quantities of fluids
- Endoscopy exam within 24 to 72 hours to assess esophagus

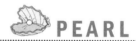

Burns of mouth *correlate poorly* with the degree of burn in the esophagus.

HYDROCARBONS

Agents
- Kerosene, charcoal lighter fluid and gas

Manifestations
- **Aspiration pneumonia**
- Acute respiratory distress syndrome
- Mild CNS depression
- Fever
- Leukocytosis
- Bilateral diffuse infiltrates on chest radiograph

Treatment
- Close monitoring for respiratory symptoms (chest x-ray)

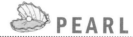

Pneumonitis may be delayed by 12 to 24 hours and coughing may be the first sign of pneumonitis.

IRON

Toxic Dose
- 20 mg/kg and higher of elemental iron

Phases

PHASE I (WITHIN 6 HOURS)
- Gastrointestinal symptoms
    - Vomiting
    - Pain
    - Diarrhea

Ingestions *continued*

IRON *continued*

PHASE II (6–24 HOURS)
- Decrease of GI symptoms and apparent improvement

PHASE III (> 24 HOURS)
- Hepatotoxicity
- Metabolic acidosis
- Coagulopathy
- Cardiovascular collapse/shock

PHASE IV (2–4 WEEKS)
- GI obstruction due to **pyloric stenosis**

Management
- Careful history to estimate amount of iron ingested
- Gastric lavage
- Whole bowel irrigation
- Iron levels at 4 hours postingestion
- Chelation with IV **deferoxamine**

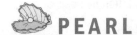 **PEARL**

Charcoal does not absorb iron effectively.

ACETAMINOPHEN

Toxic Dose
- >150 mg/kg

Stages

STAGE I (WITHIN 12–24 HOURS)
- Gastrointestinal symptoms
    —Vomiting
    —Anorexia
    —Diarrhea

STAGE II (24–48 HOURS)
- Right upper quadrant pain
- Liver enzymes begin to increase

STAGE III (72–96 HOURS)
- Hepatotoxicity
- Peak liver function abnormalities

STAGE IV (4 DAYS–2 WEEKS)
- Resolution or complete liver failure

Management
- Careful history
- Gastric lavage/activated charcoal
- Draw levels at 4 hours postingestion
- Therapy with **N-acetylcysteine** based on nomogram

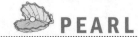 **PEARL**

If patient presents more than 6 to 8 hours after ingestion, give loading dose of N-acetylcysteine and check acetaminophen level. Never delay treatment while waiting for acetaminophen level.

Ingestion Antidotes

TOXIN	ANTIDOTE
Methanol	Ethanol
Beta-blockers	Glucagon
Calcium channel blockers	Calcium
Digitalis	Digoxin-specific antibodies
Ethanol	Dialysis
Lead	Dimercaprol (BAL) Edetate calcium-disodium (EDTA) Oral succimer (DMSA)
Methemoglobinemia	Methylene blue
Cyanide	Amyl nitrite
Phenothiazines	Benzotropine
Isoniazid	Pyridoxine
Jimson weed	Physostigmine
Warfarin	Vitamin K
Ethylene glycol	Dialysis

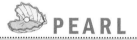

PEARL

Ethylene glycol toxic ingestions will have **calcium oxalate crystals** in the urine.

Abuse

SEXUAL ABUSE
■ Culture of *Neisseria gonorrhoeae* is **definitive of sexual abuse**

PHYSICAL ABUSE
■ Fractures more likely to be intentional:
  - "Bucket handle" metaphyseal fractures
  - Spiral fractures
  - Multiple skull fractures
  - Rib fractures
  - Posterior parietal fractures
  - Spinous process factures
  - Multiple fractures with different stages of healing
■ Burns that occur in perineum and "stocking-glove" distribution are associated with an intentional burn
■ **Family history of abuse** is the risk factor most consistently associated with abuse
■ Physical abuse is more likely to occur with children with chronic medical conditions and mental retardation
■ A work-up for abuse must be done if **retinal hemorrhages** are found on exam
■ Work-up for abuse is a skeletal survey and/or a bone scan

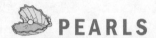 **PEARLS**

Chlamydia trachomatis can be transmitted vertically from mother to child during birth and remain until 3 years of age.

Anogenital warts/laryngeal papillomas appearing during the first year of life can be secondary to perinatal acquisition.

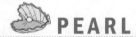 **PEARL**

Cultural therapies, including coin rubbing and cupping, are *not physical abuse*.

Concussion

Definition

Traumatically induced alteration in the level of consciousness

Grades and Recommendations

GRADE I
- **Transient confusion** without amnesia or loss of consciousness
- Athletes should be removed from game and examined every 5 minutes for development of postconcussion symptoms
- If no symptoms develop, athlete can return to game in 15 to 20 minutes

GRADE II
- Transient confusion **with amnesia** and no loss of consciousness
- Athletes should be removed from event
- Return to sport after 1 full week without symptoms

GRADE III
- Concussion with **loss of consciousness**
- Athletes should be transported to hospital for evaluation
- Return to sport after 2 full weeks without symptoms if loss of consciousness was prolonged (minutes or longer) or in 1 week if loss of consciousness was short (seconds)

Mechanical Ventilation

Intubation Tube Size (Inner Diameter)

(age in years $+$ 16) /4

Ventilator Adjustments

POSITIVE END-EXPIRATORY PRESSURE (PEEP)
- Improves **oxygenation**
- Recruits alveoli
- Used for pulmonary edema and ARDS
- Decreases venous return and cardiac output

VENTILATION RATE
- Affects alveolar **ventilation**
- Increases in ventilation rate result in decreased CO_2
- Decreases in ventilation rate result in increased CO_2

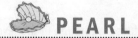

PEARL

Lidocaine, naloxone, epinephrine and atropine can be given via the intubation tube.

Foreign-Body Ingestion

Incidence

Peak occurrence is from 6 months to 3 years
Coins are the most common foreign body ingested

Management

ESOPHAGEAL:
- Asymptomatic esophageal foreign bodies should be removed if they fail to advance into the stomach in 24 hours
- Presence of foreign body in esophagus for more than 24 hours can result in perforation, TE fistula or stricture formation
- Batteries and pennies should be **removed immediately**

STOMACH:
- Batteries in the stomach usually pass; monitor progression with radiographs
- If battery in stomach for more than 48 hours, endoscopic removal is required

Recommendations for Avulsion of Teeth

1. Find the tooth.
2. Rinse tooth (do not touch the root or scrub tooth).
3. Insert tooth into socket.
4. If tooth cannot be inserted, place into milk. Older children can hold tooth in oral cavity (space between lip and teeth).
5. Go directly to dentist.

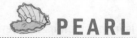

PEARL

Must prevent tooth from drying out; also avoid placing in water.

REFERENCES

1. Fleisher G, Ludwig S: Textbook of Pediatric Emergency Medicine, 4th edition, Philadelphia, Lippincott, Williams & Wilkins, 2000.

2. Behrman R, Kliegman R, Jenson H: Nelson Textbook of Pediatrics, 17th edition, Philadelphia, W.B. Saunders, 2003.

3. McMillan J, DeAngelis C, Feigin R, Warshaw J: Oski's Pediatrics—Principles and Practice, 3rd edition, Philadelphia, Lippincott, Williams & Wilkins, 1999.

4. Rudolph C, Rudolph A, Hostetter M, Lister G, Siegel N: Rudolph's Pediatrics, 21st edition, New York, McGraw-Hill, 2002.

Hyperthyroidism—Graves' Disease

Pathophysiology
- Thyroid-stimulating antibodies
- Crosses placenta, causing neonatal Graves' disease

Manifestations
- Jitteriness/tremor
- Tachycardia
- Fatigue
- Weight loss/increased appetite
- Moody/emotional
- **Exophthalmos**
- Lid lag (classic finding)

Labs

Decreased TSH
- Elevated thyroxine (T_4) and free T_4
- Elevated T_3 and free T_3
- Thyroid-stimulating antibodies

Treatment
- Propylthiouracil or methimazole
- Beta-blocker
- Surgery (used when refractory to medical treatment)

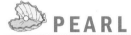 **PEARL**

McCune-Albright syndrome presents with hyperthyroidism, precocious puberty, polyostotic fibrosis, dysplasia and café-au-lait spots

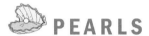 **PEARLS**

Thyroid-binding globulin increases with pregnancy, oral estrogens and during the newborn period. Patients are **euthyroid**, with lab values of elevated T_4, T_3 but a *normal free T_4*.

Subacute thyroiditis (Hashimoto's thyroiditis) can present with hyperthyroidism but the radioactive iodine uptake is *low/absent*, whereas radioactive iodine is elevated in Graves' disease.

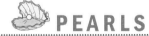 **PEARLS**

Neonatal Graves' disease can present with cardiac decompensation and is treated with propylthiouracil and beta-blockers. It usually resolves over the first several months of life.

Propylthiouracil is the preferred medication to be used during pregnancy.

SIADH

Etiology

- Meningitis/encephalitis
- Head trauma
- Guillain-Barré syndrome
- Brain tumors
- Positive airway ventilation
- Pneumonia
- Medications
  - **Vincristine/vinblastine**
  - Clofibrate
  - Cyclophosphamide
  - Chlorpropamide

Labs

- **High urine osmolarity** (250–1400 mosm/cc)
- **High urine sodium** (> 20 mEq/L)
- Hyponatremia

Treatment

- Fluid restriction (800–1000 ml/m^2/day)
- Replace urine losses of sodium
- Hyponatremic seizures: treated with **hypertonic 3% saline**
- Democlocycline (for chronic SIADH)

Diabetes Insipidus

Etiology

CENTRAL

- Craniopharyngiomas (**calcifications** on x-ray/MRI)
- Trauma (basilar skull fractures)
- Idiopathic
- Sarcoidosis
- Histoplasmosis

RENAL

- Drugs (**lithium**)
- X-linked recessive disease

Labs

- **Low urine specific gravity** (1.001–1.010)
- **Low urine osmolarity** (50–300 mosm/cc)
- Hypernatremia

Diagnosis

CENTRAL

- Low serum arginine vasopressin (AVP [ADH])
- DDAVP intranasally **increases** urine osmolarity
- Water deprivation *does not* increase urine osmolarity

RENAL

- High serum arginine vasopressin (AVP [ADH])
- DDAVP **does not increase urine** osmolarity
- Water deprivation *does not* increase urine osmolarity

Treatment

- Central—DDAVP
- Renal—adequate fluids and thiazide diuretics

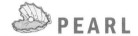

PEARL

Presents with polydipsia and polyuria; must differentiate from primary polydipsia.

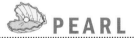

PEARL

In patients with primary polydipsia, the water deprivation *increases* the urine osmolarity.

Short Stature

FAMILIAL SHORT STATURE

Growth Pattern

- Deceleration of linear growth during the first 2 to 3 years of life
- Will then experience normal growth BUT
- Below or parallel to the fifth percentile during the prepubertal years
- Final height is *appropriate for parental heights*

Puberty

- Occurs at **expected** chronologic age

Bone Age

- **Equal** to chronologic age
- **Equal** to the height age

CONSTITUTIONAL DELAY OF GROWTH IN ADOLESCENCE ("LATE BLOOMERS")

Growth Pattern

- Deceleration of linear growth during the first 2 to 3 years of life
- Will then experience a normal growth BUT
- Below or parallel to the fifth percentile until the pre-pubertal years
- Final adult height is within the *normal range*

Puberty

- **Delayed**

Bone Age

- **Delayed** from chronologic age ($>$ 2 years)
- **Equal** to the height age

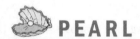 **PEARL**

Rare causes of growth deficiency include **Turner syndrome**, growth hormone deficiency, Cushing's disease, emotional deprivation, Silver-Russell syndrome (curved fifth fingers, hemihypertropy and triangular facies) and chronic illness (i.e., cystic fibrosis and hypothyroidism).

Congenital Adrenal Hyperplasia (21-Hydroxylase Deficiency)

Inheritance
- Autosomal recessive

Defect
- 21-hydroxylase deficiency (90%)
- Impaired aldosterone and cortisol production

Manifestations

SALT WASTING (75%)
- Females have ambiguous genitalia
  - Clitoromegaly
  - Fusion of labial folds/ruggae on labia
- Males phenotypically normal
- **Dehydration/shock develop at 2 to 4 weeks**

VIRILIZING (25%)
- Females born with ambiguous genitalia
- Males normal anatomy
  - Initially tall for age/advanced bone age
  - However, adult height compromised
  - Undergo precocious puberty

Labs
- **Hyponatremia**
- **Hyperkalemia**
- Metabolic acidosis

Diagnosis
- Elevated 17-hydroxyprogesterone (also in amniotic fluid)

Therapy
- Cortisol
- Mineralocorticoid

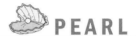 **PEARL**

Congenital adrenal hyperplasia rarely can present with female virilization in childhood; however one must also strongly consider adrenocortical tumors in these patients.

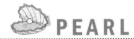 **PEARL**

Pregnancy management of woman with potential defect:
1. Initiate oral dexamethasone as soon as pregnancy detected.
2. At 10 weeks, a chorionic villus sampling is done with 21-hydroxylase genotyping.
3. If defect present, dexamethasone is stopped in males (since no risk of virilization) and continued in females until delivery.

Addison Disease

Pathophysiology
- Inadequate secretion of cortisol, aldosterone or both

Etiology

CONGENITAL
- Adrenal hypoplasia
- Adrenal hemorrhage

PRIMARY ACQUIRED
- **Autoimmune** (most common)
- Hemorrhage
- Amyloidosis
- Infection
  - Histoplasmosis
  - TB
  - Ischemic infarction with sepsis
  - Waterhouse-Friderichsen syndrome

Manifestations
Diffuse hyperpigmentation
- Salt craving
- Hypotension
- Weakness/malaise

Labs
- **Hyponatremia**
- **Hyperkalemia**
- Metabolic acidosis

Diagnosis
- Low serum cortisol
- Cortisol *unresponsive* to ACTH (ACTH stimulation test)
- **Elevated ACTH**

Treatment
- Glucocorticoids
- Mineralocorticoids

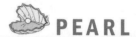

PEARL

"Secondary" adrenal insufficiency is due to ACTH deficiency from pituitary tumor, craniopharyngioma or chronic steroid therapy.

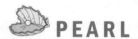

PEARL

Addison's crisis occurs with illness, surgery, trauma and results in fever, vomiting and dehydration/shock.

Diabetes Mellitus (DKA)

Presentation

- Vomiting
- Weight loss
- Polyuria
- Polydipsia
- Polyphagia
- Rapid deep breathing (Kussmaul)

Labs

- Hypoglycemia
- Metabolic acidosis
- Normal or hyperkalemia (patient is actually hypokalemic)

Treatment

- Bolus with 0.9% normal saline
- Intravenous insulin at 0.1 U/kg/h
- 5% dextrose added to IV fluids when glucose is 250 to 350 mg/dl

Complications

Cerebral Edema
- Occurs 6 to 12 hours after treatment started
- Presents with headache, lethargy, pupil abnormalities, elevated BP
- Treatment with mannitol

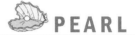

PEARL

Patients will have "fruity" breath smell.

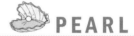

PEARL

Must address hypovolemic dehydration initially with IV fluid bolus of *isotonic* 0.9% normal saline.

Diabetes Mellitus Pearls

- Type I diabetes mellitus is associated with HLA DR3 and DR4
- Compliance of medications can be checked via hemoglobin A_1C
- *Dawn phenomenon* is a normal event and is due to the waning effects of the nighttime insulin dose. Treatment is increasing the nighttime insulin dose.
- *Somogyi phenomenon* occurs with insulin-induced hypoglycemia that results with nightmares, sweating and subsequent early morning **hyperglycemia**. Treatment is decreasing the nighttime insulin dose.
- Exercise increases glucose metabolism. Patients need to increase carbohydrate ingestion prior to exercise, and insulin may need to be decreased.
- Diagnostic Criteria
  Symptoms plus a random glucose $\geq$ 200 mg/dl
  or
  Fasting plasma glucose $\geq$ 126 mg/dl
  or
  2-hour plasma glucose (oral glucose tolerance test) $\geq$ 200 mg/dl

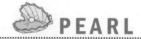

PEARL

To distinguish between the *dawn phenomenon* and the *Somogyi phenomenon,* measure glucose at 3 AM, 4 AM and 7 AM. *Somogyi phenomenon* will have a **low value** (< 60 mg/dl) at 3 AM and 4 AM and a **high value** at 7 AM. *Dawn phenomenon* will have **normal** blood glucose levels (> 80 mg/dl) at 3 AM and 4 AM and a **high value** at 7 AM.

Thyroid Nodules

"HOT" THYROID NODULES

"Hot" nodules (hyperfunctioning) on a radionucleotide scan are more likely to be **benign** with a differential diagnosis of:

- Adenomas (follicular—most common)
- Thyroiditis
- Thyrotoxicosis

"COLD" THYROID NODULES

"Cold" nodules on a radionucleotide scan are more likely to be **malignant** or non-thyroid tissue with a differential diagnosis of:

- Papillary thyroid carcinoma
  - Most common cause of childhood thyroid cancer
  - Good prognosis
  - Slow growth with local spread
- Medullary thyroid carcinoma
  - Associated with multiple endocrine neoplasia syndromes

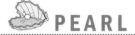
PEARL

All cold nodules should be **biopsied.**

REFERENCES

1. Shah B, Laude T: Atlas of Pediatric Clinical Diagnosis, 1st edition, Philadelphia, W.B. Saunders, 2000.

2. Behrman R, Kliegman R, Jenson H: Nelson Textbook of Pediatrics, 17th edition, Philadelphia, W.B. Saunders, 2003.

3. McMillan J, DeAngelis C, Feigin R, Warshaw J: Oski's Pediatrics—Principles and Practice, 3rd edition, Philadelphia, Lippincott, Williams & Wilkins, 1999.

4. Rudolph C, Rudolph A, Hostetter M, Lister G, Siegel N: Rudolph's Pediatrics, 21st edition, New York, McGraw-Hill, 2002.

5. AAP Red Book 2000, 25th edition, 2000.

ETHICS

Definitions

MATURE MINOR
- Adolescents older than 14 years of age who understand the risks and benefits of services being provided and can give informed consent

EMANCIPATED MINOR
- Adolescents 16 years of age or older who are any of the following:
  - Married
  - Have joined the armed forces
  - Living on their own and managing their own finances
  - Pregnant (usually given status of emancipated minor)

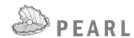

Involuntary urine testing of adolescents violates their legal rights of informed consent in a competent patient.

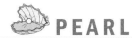

Emancipated minors do not need parental consent for health care services.

Ethical Pearls

FOREGOING LIFE-SUSTAINING MEDICAL TREATMENT
- Physicians and parents should give **great weight** to clearly expressed views of children regarding life-sustaining medical treatment *regardless* of the legal matters.
- Mature and emancipated minor may refuse unwanted medical treatment.

EMERGENCY TREATMENT
- Physicians do not need parental consent to treat.
- Does not have to be life-threatening to be treated without consent (i.e., lacerations).
- Preadolescents may not refuse medical care.

INFORMED CONSENT AND ADOLESCENT PATIENTS
- If parents and adolescent patient want unconventional therapy (i.e., herb therapy for leukemia), physician should consider a court order for conventional treatments.
- If Jehovah Witness adolescent wants blood transfusion over parent's objection, the patient's interest should prevail.

REFUSAL OF TREATMENT (YOUNG CHILDREN/PARENT REFUSAL)
- If **prognosis is good**, courts orders will nearly always be granted (i.e., blood transfusion following trauma in Jehovah's Witness).
- If **prognosis is poor**, courts typically side with parents.
- Physicians have no legal duty to insist on treatment that will delay death in a terminal illness.

REFERENCES

1. Rudolph C, Rudolph A, Hostetter M, Lister G, Siegel N: Rudolph's Pediatrics, 21st edition, New York, McGraw-Hill, 2002.

2. Behrman R, Kliegman R, Jenson H: Nelson's Textbook of Pediatrics, 17th edition, Philadelphia, W.B. Saunders, 2003.

GASTROENTEROLOGY

Hematemesis

Pathophysiology

- Bleeding *proximal* to the ligament of Treitz
- Bright red or coffee ground emesis

Common Causes

NEWBORN

- Swallowed maternal blood
- Gastritis
- Peptic ulcer disease
- Bleeding diathesis

INFANTS/YOUNG CHILDREN

- Esophagitis
- Peptic ulcer disease

OLDER CHILDREN/ADOLESCENTS

- Esophagitis
- Peptic ulcer disease
- Gastritis
- Esophageal varices
- Mallory-Weiss tear

Diagnosis

- Upper gastrointestinal endoscopy

Differential Diagnosis of Rectal Bleeding

Newborn

- Vitamin K deficiency
- Swallowed maternal blood (Apt-Downey test to identify fetal vs. maternal blood)
- Cow's milk allergy
- Infectious diarrhea

Infant to 2 Years of Age

- **Anal fissure** (common)
- Meckel's diverticulum
- Milk allergy
- Infectious diarrhea
- Intussusception

Two years to Preschool

- Infectious diarrhea
- Polyp
- Intussusception
- Anal fissure
- Hemolytic-uremic syndrome
- Henoch-Schönlein purpura syndrome

Preschool to Adolescence

- **Polyp** (common)
- Inflammatory bowel disease
- Infectious diarrhea
- Ulcer
- Varices

Inflammatory Bowel Disease

	CROHN'S DISEASE	ULCERATIVE COLITIS
Location:	Mouth to anus	**Colon only**
Pathology:	**Transmural inflammation** Discontinuous/**"skip areas"** Fibrosis/strictures **Perianal fistulas** Granulomas	Mucosal inflammation Crypt abscesses Diffuse involvement
Manifestations:	Nonbloody diarrhea Crampy abdominal pain Poor growth Weight loss Feelings of fullness Fevers Strictures	**Rectal bleeding** Bloody diarrhea Fevers Tenesmus Abdominal pain
Extra-intestinal Sequelae:	Arthritis **Erythema nodosum** Hepatitis Uveitis/iritis **Oral ulcers** Perianal lesions	**Increased colon cancer** Pyoderma gangrenosum Cholangitis Uveitis/iritis Ankylosing spondylitis Hepatitis
Radiologic Findings:	**"String sign"** Skip lesions Longitudinal ulcers	Decreased colon haustrations **"Collar button" ulcers** **"Lead pipe" colon**
Treatment:	Sulfasalazine Corticosteroids Anti-TNF alpha 6-Mercaptopurine Methotrexate Azathioprine Surgery	Sulfasalazine Corticosteroids Cyclosporine **Surgery—curative**

AAP Guidelines for Management of Gastroenteritis

- Oral rehydration using a balanced glucose-electrolyte is the preferred treatment for dehydration up to 9%.
- Severe dehydration (> 10%), should be treated with intravenous therapy.
- Intravenous fluids should be used for children with ileus, who are unconscious, and in whom vomiting precludes adequate fluid retention.
- Regular feedings should be continued in children with mild dehydration.
- Breast-feeding should be *continued*.
- There is **no indication** for clear fluids, BRAT diet, lactose-restricted diets or a 24-hour bowel rest period.
- Children should be fed age-appropriate diets as soon as rehydrated.
- Pharmacologic agents (loperamide, opiates and anticholinergic agents) should not be used to treat acute diarrhea.
- Typical oral rehydration solutions used in the USA (i.e., Pedialyte) have 45 mmol/L of sodium and 25 gm/L of carbohydrate; WHO/UNICEF solutions contain 90 mmol/L of sodium and 20 gm/L of carbohydrate.
- Parents should not use low electrolyte/high carbohydrate (hypertonic) solutions such as colas, apple juice or chicken broth for oral rehydration.
- *Lactobacillus*-containing compounds and bismuth subsalicylate are not recommended for treating acute diarrhea.

Chronic Nonspecific Diarrhea (Toddlers' Diarrhea)

Epidemiology
- Most **common** cause of chronic diarrhea of childhood

Age Range
- 6–20 months

Pathogenesis
- Secondary to altered gastrointestinal motility
- Accelerated transit of contents through the GI tract

Diet History
- Low fat intake
- Increased intake of carbohydrates (often apple juice)

Stools Pattern
- Two to ten a day
- Malodorous
- Watery/brown
- Contain mucus or **undigested food particles**

Treatment
- **High-fat, low carbohydrate diet**
- Modest fluid restriction
- Minimize sorbitol-containing drinks (i.e., apple juice)

Prognosis
- Resolves spontaneously by 40 months of age

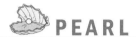
PEARL

Despite altered transit time, children have normal adsorption, growth and height gains.

Hirschsprung Disease

Pathophysiology

■ Failure of ganglion on myenteric plexus to migrate in colon

Manifestations

■ Constipation
■ Poor feeding
■ Vomiting
■ Abdominal distention

Radiography

BARIUM ENEMA

■ **Transition zone** between narrowed abnormal distal end and dilated normal proximal end

Diagnosis

■ Rectal biopsy

Treatment

■ Surgery

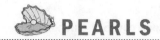

PEARLS

Must be considered in children who do not pass meconium in first 24 hours of life or who need rectal stimulation to induce bowel movements.

Celiac Disease

Epidemiology

- Presents between 6 months and 2 years of age

Pathophysiology

- Immunologic response to gluten
- Small bowel manifestations
    —Villous atrophy
    —Crypt hyperplasia

Associated Foods

- Wheat, rye, barley and possibly oats

Manifestations

- Failure to thrive
- Abdominal distention
- Diarrhea/foul-smelling stools
- **Muscle wasting (extremities/buttocks)**

Associated Diseases

- IgA deficiency
- Diabetes mellitus
- Down syndrome

Diagnosis

- IgA endomysial antibody
- Small bowel biopsy

Treatment

- Lifelong strict gluten-free diet

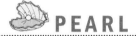

PEARL

Corn and rice are not associated with disease.

Pyloric Stenosis

Epidemiology

- Males:females (4:1)
- Higher in first-born males
- Higher risk with history of maternal pyloric stenosis

Manifestations

- Peak occurrence is 2 to 4 weeks of age
- **Nonbilious projectile** emesis
- **Olive-sized mass** in epigastic area
- Visible peristaltic waves may be seen

Diagnosis

- Abdominal ultrasound reveals hypertrophic pylorus

Treatment

- Initially, nasogastric tube
- Electrolyte/fluid management
- Surgery

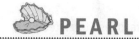

PEARL

Hypokalemic, hypochloremic metabolic alkalosis is seen secondary to severe dehydration.

REFERENCES

1. Rudolph C, Rudolph A, Hostetter M, Lister G, Siegel N: Rudolph's Pediatrics, 21st edition, New York, McGraw Hill, 2002.

2. Behrman R, Kliegman R, Jenson H: Nelson's Textbook of Pediatrics, 17th edition, Philadelphia, W.B. Saunders, 2003.

3. McMillan J, deAngelis C, Feigin R, Warshaw J: Oski's Pediatrics—Principles and Practice, 3rd edition, Philadelphia, Lippincott, Williams & Wilkins, 1999.

4. Clinical Practice Guidelines of the American Academy of Pediatrics, 1999.

GENETICS

CHAPTER

11

Glycogen Storage Diseases

TYPE I—VON GIERKE DISEASE

Deficiency
- Hepatic glucose-6-phosphatase (autosomal recessive)

Manifestations
- Hypoglycemia (neonatal)
- Hepatosplenomegaly
- **"Doll's facies"**

Labs
- Lactic acidosis
- Ketones without reducing substances
- Elevated triglycerides

Treatment
- Nocturnal infusion of glucose with infants
- Raw corn starch in water for older children

TYPE II—POMPE DISEASE (INFANTILE)

Deficiency
- Alpha-glucosidase (autosomal recessive)

Manifestations
- Profound muscle weakness/floppy baby
- Cardiomegaly
- **Short PR interval**

Labs
- Elevated serum creatine kinase

Prognosis
- Death in the first year of life

Glycogen Storage Diseases *continued*

TYPE V—MCARDLE DISEASE

Deficiency
- Muscle phosphorylase (autosomal recessive)

Manifestations
- **Exercise intolerance** with severe cramps
- Begins in adolescence
- Burgundy urine after exercise

Labs
- Elevated creatine kinase
- Mild hypoglycemia

Treatment
- Avoidance of strenuous exercise

Down Syndrome

TRISOMY 21 (47 CHROMOSOMES)—95% OF CASES

Inheritance

- Nondisjunction at chromosome 21

Risk in Future Pregnancies

- 1 to 2%

TRANSLOCATION (46 CHROMOSOMES)

Inheritance

- Translocation between chromosomes 21 and 13, 14 or 15
- 75% are not familial
- 25% are familial

Risk in Future Pregnancies

- 15 to 100%

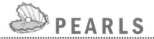

PEARLS

Incidence increases with **maternal age** and prenatally associated with a *decreased* alpha-fetoprotein, decreased estradiol and *increased* HCG.

Elevated alpha-fetoprotein is associated with anencephaly, open spinabifida, ventral wall defects or an incorrect gestation age.

Down Syndrome

Manifestations

CARDIAC DISEASE (50%)
- **Endocardial cushion defects**, ASD or VSD
  - evaluation before 6 months in all cases

MUSCULOSKELETAL
- Prenatal nuchal pad thickening
- Decreased tone
- Simian crease
- Flat occiput/flat facies
- Atlantoaxial instability
  - Screen via lateral cervical spines during life

ENDOCRINE
- Diabetes
- Autoimmune hypothyroidism
  - Periodic thyroid screening

CENTRAL NERVOUS SYSTEM
- Decreased IQ: 40 to 70

OPHTHALMOLOGY
- Speckled iris ("**Brushfield spots**")
- Cataracts/myopia
  - Ophthalmology exam at 4 years of age

HEMATOLOGIC
- 30% will develop **transient abnormal myelopoiesis**, which usually resolves in the first 3 months of life
- 20% will develop leukemia

GASTROINTESTINAL
- Duodenal atresia (maternal polyhydramnios)
  - X-ray shows "double-bubble sign"

Achondroplasia

Inheritance

- Autosomal dominant (FGFR3 gene mutation)

Manifestations

- Dwarfism
- Macrocephaly
- Frontal bossing
- Proximal shortening of the extremities
- Depressed nasal bridge

Radiographic Findings

- Small foramen magnum
- "Trident" hand
- Shortening of limbs
- Prominent frontal bones

Complications

- Hydrocephalus—secondary to small foramen magnum
- Hypotonia (in infancy)
- Lumbar spinal stenosis
- Neurologic defects—secondary to narrow spinal canal
- Apnea—2° to cord compression at foramen magnum

Progeny Risks

If **both parents** have achondroplasia
- 25% chance of homozygous child—*fatal* in newborn
- 25% chance of normal child
- 50% chance of child with achondroplasia

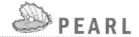

PEARL

Increased paternal age increases risk for new mutation.

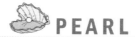

PEARL

Nearly all have **normal intelligence**.

Prader-Willi Syndrome   15

Inheritance

GENE DELETION (75% OF PATIENTS)
- Interstitial deletion of chromosome 15 (15q11-13)
- Phenomenon of "**genomic imprinting**"

UNIPARENTAL DISOMY (25% OF PATIENTS)
- Have two *normal maternally* derived chromosome 15

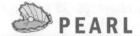

PEARL

Deletion is *paternally derived*.

Diagnosis

Fluorescent *in situ* hybridization (FISH)

Manifestations

MUSCULOSKELETAL
- Hypotonia
- Small hands and feet

GENITOURINARY
- Micropenis

GASTROINTESTINAL
- In infancy, poor feeding and **failure to thrive**
- As they age, become **hyperphagic and obese**

CENTRAL NERVOUS SYSTEM
- Mental impairment

Angelman Syndrome

Inheritance

GENE DELETION (60% OF PATIENTS)
- Interstitial deletion arm of chromosome 15 (15q11-13)
- Phenomenon of **"genomic imprinting"**

UNIPARENTAL DISOMY (40% OF PATIENTS)
- Have two normal *paternally derived* chromosome 15

Manifestations

MUSCULOSKELETAL
- Ataxic gait—**"puppet-like gait"**
- **"Clown facies"**

CENTRAL NERVOUS SYSTEM
- Severe motor/intellectual impairment
- Hyperactivity
- Microcephaly
- Seizures
- **Inappropriate laughter**

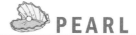

PEARL

Deletion is *maternally derived.*

Beckwith-Wiedemann Syndrome

Inheritance
- Two copies of paternally derived chromosome 11p15.5

Manifestations

ENDOCRINE
- Neonatal hypoglycemia secondary to hyperinsulinemia

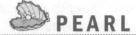

At risk for neonatal **hypoglycemic seizures.**

MUSCULOSKELETAL
- Gigantism
- Hemihypertrophy
- **Macroglossia**
- Macrosomia
- **Earlobe fissures** (classic finding)

ABDOMINAL
- Visceromegaly
- Omphalocele
- Umbilical hernia

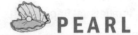

Must have serial abdominal ultrasound every 3 months until the age of 7 years and monitoring of alpha-fetoprotein (associated with Wilms' tumor and hepatoblastomas).

ONCOLOGIC
- Intra-abdominal embryonal malignancies
  - Wilms' tumor
  - Hepatoblastoma
  - Adrenal carcinoma

DiGeorge Syndrome

Inheritance
- Microdeletion of chromosome 22

Diagnosis
- Fluorescent *in situ* hybridization (FISH)

Manifestations

CARDIAC
- Interrupted aortic arch
- Truncus arteriosus
- Hypoparathyroidism
- **Hypocalcemia**

IMMUNOLOGIC
- Thymic hypoplasia
- T-cell defects
- Can be immunocompromised and need prophylactic antibiotics

FACIES
- Micrognathia
- Hypertelorism
- Low-set ears

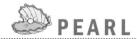

PEARL

Presents as **hypocalcemic seizures**, which are treated with IV calcium gluconate. After stabilized, treat with PO calcitriol (1,25-dihydroxy-cholecalciferol).

Wilson Disease

Inheritance

- Autosomal recessive

Manifestations

HEPATIC
- Hepatomegaly/hepatitis
- Cirrhosis

CENTRAL NERVOUS SYSTEM
- Dysarthria
- Movement disorders
- Loss of IQ/ deterioration in school performance
- Behavior changes

OPHTHALMOLOGIC
- **Kayser-Fleischer rings** (deposits of copper in iris)
  - Golden brown pigmentation in the outer crescent of the iris

HEMATOLOGIC
- Hemolysis

Labs

- **Reduced levels of plasma ceruloplasmin**
- Increased levels of nonceruloplasmin copper
- Increased urinary excretion of copper

Treatment

- Diet restriction of copper-rich foods (i.e., nuts, chocolate)
- Penicillamine (copper chelator)
- Zinc (decreases copper absorption)

Prognosis

- Variable; may need liver transplantation

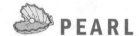

PEARL

Typically presents in late childhood or adolescence with **behavior/personality/psychiatric symptoms.**

Phenylketonuria (PKU)

Inheritance
- Autosomal recessive

Deficiency
- Phenylalanine hydroxylase *or* tetrahydrobiopterin

Excessive Metabolite
- Phenylalanine

Manifestations
- **Blond hair**
- Blue eyes
- Fair skinned
- **"Musty" odor**
- Mental retardation
- Hypertonic/hyperreflexia

Treatment

PHENYLALANINE HYDROXYLASE DEFICIENCY
- Restrict phenylalanine

TETRAHYDROBIOPTERIN DEFICIENCY
- Restrict phenylalanine
- Tetrahydrobiopterin
- Dopamine/serotonin

Pregnant Women Recommendations
- Must restrict phenylalanine. If phenylalanine levels are greater then 10 mg/dl, there is a *high risk* of:
    - Spontaneous abortion
    - Mental retardation
    - Cardiac defects
    - Low birth weights

Prognosis
- Without restriction, **severe mental retardation**

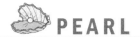

PEARL

All infants with hyperphenylalaninemia must be assessed for a **deficiency of tetrahydrobiopterin.**

Homocystinuria

Inheritance
- Autosomal recessive

Defect
- Deficiency of cystathionine beta-synthase

Manifestations

MUSCULOSKELETAL
- Tall/thin
- Scoliosis

CENTRAL NERVOUS SYSTEM
- **Mental impairment** (progressive)

OPHTHALMOLOGIC
- **Dislocated lenses** (ectopia lentis)
- Myopia

HEMATOLOGIC
- **Thromboembolism**

Diagnosis
- Confirmed by increased methionine and homocystine

Treatment
- 50% respond to pyridoxine (vitamin B$_6$)
- Folate
- Cysteine
- Low-methionine diet

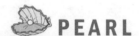 **PEARL**

Homocystinuria can have *similar* manifestations to Marfan syndrome but has mental impairment and does not have cardiac involvement.

Tay Sachs

Inheritance

■ Autosomal recessive

Enzyme Deficiency

■ beta-hexosaminidase A (lysosomal storage disease)

Manifestations

CENTRAL NERVOUS SYSTEM (STARTS BEFORE 9 MONTHS OF AGE)
■ Rapid progressive neurodegeneration
  - Children never ambulate
  - Hypotonia
  - Apathy
  - **Exaggerated startle**
  - Blindness
  - Seizures

OPHTHALMOLOGIC
■ **"Cherry-red"** spot on fundoscopic exam

Diagnosis

■ Decreased hexoaminidase in blood leukocytes

Prognosis

■ Death (usually by 5 years of age)

Prenatal Diagnosis

■ Via chorionic villus sampling or amniocentesis

VACTERL

Vertebral defects

Anal atresia

Cardiac malformations

TE Fistula

USUALLY WITH PROXIMAL ESOPHAGEAL POUCH
- Associated with **maternal polyhydramnios**
- Excessive oral secretions, choking and poor feeding

Renal anomalies

Limb anomalies

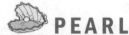 **PEARL**

Diagnose by placing nasogastric tube and checking a chest x-ray (tube will be coiled in pouch)..

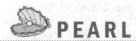 **PEARL**

Single artery umbilical cords are associated with renal anomalies, and these children may need a renal ultrasound.

Marfan Syndrome

Inheritance

- Autosomal dominant (defects of fibrillin gene)

Features

CARDIAC
- Aortic regurgitation
- Mitral regurgitation
- Mitral valve prolapse
- **Dilation of ascending aorta**

MUSCULOSKELETAL
- Tall stature
- Pectus excavatum
- Scoliosis
- Hyperextensible joints
- Arachnodactyly

OPHTHALMOLOGIC
- **Ectopia lentis**

Diagnosis

- A major feature in at least two organ systems and involvement of a third organ system

Treatment

- Beta-blockers

Risks

- At risk of **sudden death** from aortic rupture

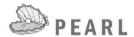 **PEARL**

Marfan syndrome can have similar manifestations to homocystinuria but has cardiac involvement without mental retardation.

Duchenne Muscular Dystrophy

Inheritance

■ X-linked recessive (mutation of the dystrophin gene)

Manifestations

MUSCULOSKELETAL
■ **Gower sign**—(the need to press on thighs to rise from floor)
■ Clumsiness/waddling gait
■ Toe-walking
■ **Pseudohypertrophy** of calves

CARDIAC
■ Cardiomyopathy

CENTRAL NERVOUS SYSTEM
■ Intellectual impairment

Labs

■ **Elevated serum creatine kinase**

Diagnosis

■ Muscle biopsy
■ Defective dystrophin by immunohistochemical staining

Treatment

■ Supportive

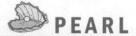

PEARL

Maternal carriers will give all sons *disease* and 50% of daughters the *gene*.

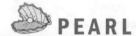

PEARL

Becker muscular dystrophy presents with similar symptoms but later and with a slower progression.

Fragile X Syndrome

Inheritance

- X-linked recessive
- Gene mutation with increased CCG/CGG triplets

Manifestations

MALES

- **Macro-orchidism** (following puberty)
- Mental retardation
- Macrocephaly
- Large ears
- Prominent brow
- Coarse facies

FEMALES

- Mental deficiencies

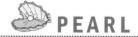

PEARL

Syndrome due to **allelic expansion**. CGG/CCG triplets can increase from one generation to the next and eventually become large enough and lead to Fragile X phenotype.

Turner Syndrome

Inheritance

- 45,X (50%)
- Mosaics: 45,X/46,XX, 45,X/46,XY or others

Manifestations

MUSCULOSKELETAL
- Prenatal nuchal pad thickening
- **Lymphedema of hands and feet** during infancy
- **Webbed neck**
- Wide-spaced nipples
- Short stature
- Low posterior hairline

CARDIOVASCULAR
- Coarctation of the aorta
- Bicuspid aortic valve
- Aortic stenosis

RENAL
- Horseshoe kidney
- Duplicated collecting system

CENTRAL NERVOUS SYSTEM
- Intelligence is normal

GYNECOLOGIC
- Gonadal dysgenesis (streak ovaries)

Diagnosis

- Karyotype

Treatment

- Growth hormone
- Estrogens
- Psychological supports

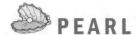

Turner syndrome must be considered in any female with short stature.

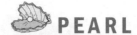

Consider as diagnosis in cases of primary amenorrhea and/or lack or sexual maturation.

Klinefelter Syndrome

Karyotype

■ 47, XXY

Manifestations

MUSCULOSKELETAL
■ Tall
■ **Gynecomastia**

UROLOGIC
■ **Small testes**
■ Infertile

CENTRAL NERVOUS SYSTEM
■ Decreased intelligence (mild)
■ Behavior problems

Treatment

■ Testosterone may be indicated at adolescence.

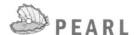

PEARL

Increases with advanced maternal age.

Trisomy 13 and 18

TRISOMY 13 (PATAU SYNDROME)

Manifestations

- Localized **scalp defects** in the parieto-occipital area
- Holoprosencephaly
- Microophthalmia
- Coloboma
- Cleft lip/palate
- Flexed fingers
- Cardiac malformations
- Severe mental retardation

TRISOMY 18 (EDWARDS SYNDROME)

Manifestations

- **Closed fist**
  - Second finger overlaps the third
  - Fourth finger overlaps the fifth
- **Rockerbottom feet**
- Microcephaly
- Cardiac malformations
- Renal anomalies
- Severe mental retardation

Miscellaneous Syndromes with Hearing Loss

WAARDENBURG
- **White forelock**
- Hypopigmentation of the fundi
- Partial albinism
- Sensorineural hearing loss (unilateral or bilateral)
- Hypertelorism

USHER
- **Retinitis pigmentosa**
- Sensorineural hearing loss

STICKLER
- Flattened facial profile
- Cleft palate
- Myopia
- Retinal detachment
- Conductive/sensorineural hearing loss

GOLDENHAR
- Facial asymmetry
- **Ear anomalies (external and internal)**
- Conductive hearing loss
- Vertebral anomalies

CONGENITAL RUBELLA SYNDROME
- Sensorineural deafness
- Cataracts
- Intrauterine growth retardation
- "Blueberry muffin" lesions

Galactosemia

Inheritance

■ Autosomal recessive

Enzyme Deficiency

■ Galactose-1-phosphate uridyl transferase

Presentation

■ Presents in neonate, days to weeks after fed glucose

Manifestations

GASTROINTESTINAL
■ **Vomiting**
■ Jaundice
■ Hepatomegaly
■ Failure to thrive

CENTRAL NERVOUS SYSTEM
■ Lethargy
■ CNS/neurologic depression
■ Seizures

OPHTHALMOLOGIC
■ **Cataracts**

Labs

■ Reducing substances in urine (via Clinitest)

Diagnosis

■ Deficient galactose-1-phosphate uridyl transferase in RBC
■ Increased galactose-1-phosphate in RBC

Treatment

■ Restriction of galactose in diet

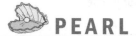

PEARL

Associated with **gram-negative sepsis** with poor response to antibiotics until appropriate dietary therapy initiated.

Osteogenesis Imperfecta

Inheritance
- Autosomal dominant

Manifestations
- **Fragile bones/fractures**
- **Blue sclera**
- **Early deafness** (sensorineural)

Types

TYPE I (MILD)
- Subtype A: normal dentition
- Subtype B: dentinogenesis imperfecta
- Joint laxity
- Fractures decrease after puberty
- Blue sclera persist

TYPE II (PERINATAL LETHAL)
- Numerous intrauterine fractures
- **Stillborn** or death in the newborn period

TYPE III (PROGRESSIVE DEFORMING)
- Severest nonlethal form
- Sclera can lighten with age
- Usually have **intrauterine fractures**
- Wormian bones (undermineralized calvarium)

TYPE IV (MODERATELY SEVERE)
- Subtype A: normal dentition
- Subtype B: dentinogenesis imperfecta
- **Bowing** of the lower long bones
- Attain ambulation
- Sclera can lighten with age

Diagnosis
- Collagen biochemical studies with fibroblasts

Autosomal Dominant Disorders

ALAGILLE SYNDROME

Cholestasis
Elevated conjugated bilirubin
Paucity of interlobar bile ducts
Butterfly vertebrae
Peripheral pulmonary stenosis

VON HIPPEL-LINDAU

Cavernous hemangiomas
Hemangioblastomas
Adenomas
Renal cell carcinomas
Pheocytochromas

GILBERT'S DISEASE

Elevated unconjugated bilirubin
Treated with phenobarbital

FAMILIAL HYPERCHOLESTEREMIA

Atherosclerosis
Xanthomas

HUNTINGTON DISEASE

Atrophy of caudate nucleus
Extrapyramidal/choreiform movements
Presents > 30 years old

MYOTONIC DYSTROPHY

Myotonia/apathetic facies
Worsens each decade
Breech/arthrogryposis

ALBRIGHT HEREDITARY OSTEODYSTROPHY

Pseuodhypoparathyroidism
Short fourth/fifth metacarpals
Hypocalcemia
Seizures

EHLERS-DANLOS

Hyperextensibility of joints
Hyperextensibility of skin
Poor wound healing

CYCLIC NEUTROPENIA

Neutropenia every 21 to 28 days
Oral ulcers
Clostridium perfringens sepsis
Treat with G-CSF therapy

APERT SYNDROME

Syndactyly of toes/hand digits
Premature suture fusion
Progressive calcification of bones

CHARCOT-MARIE-TOOTH DISEASE

Common cause of **peripheral neuropathy**
Asymptomatic until late childhood
Easily trip/clumsy (foot drop)
Leg muscle atrophy (stork-like legs)
Normal intelligence

CROUZON SYNDROME

Craniofacial dysostosis
Premature craniosynostosis
Exophthalmos
Frontal bossing

GARDNER SYNDROME

Multiple intestinal polyps
Central nervous system tumors
Hepatoblastomas
Osteomas
Pigmented ocular fundus
Mutation of *APC* gene
Supernumerary teeth
Polyps are premalignant; aggressive surgery

GILLES DE LA TOURETTE

Multiple tics
Shouting obscene words
Grunting/twitching
Treat with haloperidol

OSLER-WEBER-RENDU SYNDROME

Telangiectasis:
—Lips   —Lungs
—Tongue   —Brain
—GI tract
Bleeding (nose/GI common)

ADULT POLYCYSTIC KIDNEY DISEASE

Bilateral renal cysts
Presents > 30 years old

TREACHER COLLINS SYNDROME

Hypoplastic mandible
Deafness

Autosomal Recessive Disorders

PYRIDOXINE DEFICIENCY

Seizures
Treat with vitamin B_6

CRIGLER NAJJAR

Unconjugated bilirubin
Becomes elevated as neonate

UREA CYCLE DEFICITS

Elevated ammonia
No ketones

POLYCYSTIC KIDNEY DISEASE

Bilateral renal masses

AUTOIMMUNE POLYENDOCRINOPATHY

Hypoparathyroidism
Alopecia
Addison disease
Mucocutaneous candidiasis
Pernicious anemia

FANCONI

Brown pigmentation
Pancytopenia
Aplasia of thumbs
Short stature
Need bone marrow transplant

NEPHROPATHIC CYSTINOSIS

Corneal opacities
Fanconi syndrome
Cysteine crystals in cornea
Failure to thrive
Treatment: cysteamine

MEDIUM-CHAIN ACYL-COA DEHYDROGENASE DEFICIENCY

Presents in first 2 years of life
Hypoketotic hypoglycemia
Elevated ammonia
Clinical only in fasting state
Treatment: acyl carnitine

SHWACHMAN-DIAMOND SYNDROME

Neutropenia
Pancreatic insufficiency
Malabsorption/steatorrhea
Sepsis

SMITH-LEMLI-OPITZ SYNDROME

Ptosis of eyelids
Hypospadias/cryptorchidism
Syndactyly of second/third toes
Elevated 7-dehydrocholesterol
Low cholesterol

ABETALIPOPROTEINEMIA

Severe fat malabsorption
Failure to thrive
Ataxia around 10 years old
Need vitamin A/D/E/K
Acanthocytes (spiny projections on RBCs)

COCKAYNE SYNDROME

Birdlike facies
Dwarfism
Premature senility
Photosensitivity
Mental retardation

BLOOM SYNDROME

Facial telangiectasia (butterfly distribution)
Photosensitivity
Increased malignancy (leukemia)

DUBIN-JOHNSON SYNDROME

Conjugated hyperbilirubinemia
Hepatocytes contain black pigment
Abnormal gallbladder

FARBER SYNDROME

Deficiency of acid ceramidase
Nodules over joints
Painful joint swelling
Hoarseness

FRIEDREICH ATAXIA

Ataxia develops around 10 years old
Explosive dysarthric speech
Loss of vibration/position sense
Posterior column degeneration
High-arched feet
Hypertrophic cardiomyopathy

Autosomal Recessive Disorders *continued*

FRUCTOSE INTOLERANCE SYNDROME

Deficiency of fructose 1,6-bisPO$_4$
  aldolase
Healthy until fructose ingested
Fructose found in juices, fruit, cereals
Symptoms resemble galactosemia
Vomiting, hepatomegaly, jaundice
Reducing substances found in urine
Avoid sucrose, fructose and sorbitol

GLANZMANN THROMBASTHENIA

Defective platelet aggregation
Normal platelet count/smear
Prolonged bleeding time

GAUCHER'S DISEASE

Glucocerebrosidase deficiency
Type I—adult (nonneuropathic)
Type II—infant (death by 2 years old)
Type III—juvenile (neuropathic)

NIEMANN-PICK DISEASE

Sphingomyelinase deficiency
Macular cherry-red spot
Hepatomegaly
Type A—infantile neuropathy

HURLER SYNDROME

α-L-iduronidase deficiency
Heparan/dermatan sulfate accumulate
Corneal clouding
Dwarfism
CNS deficits

ALKAPTONURIA

Homogentisic oxidase deficiency
Excrete homogentisic acid
Urine turns black

HARTNUP DISEASE

Defect of neutral amino acids transport
  in kidney
Aminoaciduria
**Normal urine levels of arginine,
  proline**
Fanconi has high urine levels of
  arginine, proline
Photosensitivity (pellagra-like rash
  develops)
Can be benign/asymptomatic
Treatment: nicotinic acid

ROTOR SYNDROME

Conjugated hyperbilirubinemia
Liver cells contain no black pigment

X-linked Recessive Disorders

MENKES SYNDROME

Decreased copper/ceruloplasmin
Seizures
Twisted/fractured hair
Progressive CNS deterioration

ADRENOLEUKODYSTROPHY

Peroxisomal disorder
CNS deterioration
Adrenal insufficiency
Spasticity
Blindness/deafness

HUNTER SYNDROME

L-iduronosulfate sulfatase defect
Heparan/dermatan sulfate accumulate
Dwarfism
No corneal clouding
CNS deterioration

FABRAY'S DISEASE

α-galactosidase A defects
Ceramide trihexosidase accumulates
Angiokeratomas
Burning pain
Renal failure

ORNITHINE TRANSCARBAMYLASE DEFICIENCY

Elevated ammonia
Elevated lactic acid
No ketones
Increased urine orotic acid
Respiratory alkalosis

LOWE SYNDROME

Congenital cataracts
Mental retardation
Fanconi syndrome

ECTODERMAL DYSPLASIA

Absence of sweat glands
Absent teeth/anomalous dentition
Mistaken to have fevers
Diagnosed via skin biopsy

LESCH-NYHAN DISEASE

Hypoxanthine-guanine phosphoribosyl
  transferase deficiency
Gout
Self-mutilation
Aggressive behavior

X-linked Dominant Disxorders

AICARDI SYNDROME

Lethal in males
CNS deterioration
Agenesis of corpus callosum
Profound mental deficiency

INCONTINENTIA PIGMENTI SYNDROME

Ocular problems
CNS defects (seizures, cognitive deficiencies, spasticity)
Dental anomalies
Four phases of lesions:
1. Linear streaks/vesicles on limbs/trunk
2. Verrucous plaques on limbs
3. **Hyperpigmented macular whorls** on trunk/limbs
4. Hypopigmented, hairless, anhidrotic patches on flexural areas

Miscellaneous Syndromes

ZELLWEGER

Hypotonia
High forehead
Hepatomegaly
Peroxisomal disorder
Elevated plasma long-chain fatty acids
Severe mental retardation

CORNELIA DE LANGE

Hirsuitism
Bushy eyebrows
Mental retardation

WILLIAMS

Supravalvular aortic stenosis
Elevated calcium
"Friendly" personality
Elfin facies
Stellate iris
Diagnosis: FISH

NOONAN

"Male Turner syndrome"
Pulmonic stenosis
Mental retardation
Webbed neck
Pectus excavatum

PEUTZ JEGHERS

Mucocutaneous pigmentation
Intestinal polyposis
Risk of adenocarcinomas
—Lung
—Pancreas
—Breast
—Thyroid
—Gallbladder

KARTAGENER

Immotile cilia
Sinusitis
Bronchiectasis
Situs inversus
Sterile

RILEY-DAY SYNDROME

Degenerative CNS disease
Attacks of hypertension
Transient skin blotching
Episodes of hyperpyrexia/vomiting
Insensitive to pain

AMYOTROPHIC LATERAL SCLEROSIS

Upper and lower motor neuron disease
Fibrillations/fasciculations
Lesions in anterior horn/brain
Muscle weakness/atrophy

BARTTER SYNDROME

Hypokalemic (renal losses)
Hyperplasia of juxtaglomerular
   apparatus
Metabolic alkalosis
Elevated renin/aldosterone
Normal blood pressure

CRI DU CHAT SYNDROME

Partial chromosome deletion
Cat-like cry
Microcephaly
Mental deficiency

PROGERIA SYNDROME

Premature aging
Alopecia
Atherosclerosis
Delayed teeth eruption

PIERRE ROBIN SYNDROME

Micrognathia
Arched/cleft
Tongue obstructs airway
Maintain child in prone position
30% need tracheostomy

EAGLE-BARRET SYNDROME

Prune belly syndrome
Renal/genitourinary defects

MOBIUS SYNDROME

Sixth/seventh cranial nerve palsy
Dull facies

Miscellaneous Syndromes *continued*

WEGENER'S GRANULOMATOSIS

Necrotizing granulomatous vasculitis
Kidney, upper and lower airway affected
Antibodies to PR-3 (c-ANCA)
Treatment: cyclophosphamide/steroids

KALLMANN SYNDROME

Hypogonadotropic hypogonadism
Anosmia

TESTICULAR FEMINIZATION

Receptors are resistant to testosterone
Genetically: "XY" and male
Phenotypically: female
Blind vaginal pouch, sparse pubic hair
Amenorrhea/sterile
Testes in inguinal canal or labial folds
Orchiectomy secondary to neoplastic
  risks
**Consider as diagnosis in females
  with hernias**

REFERENCES

1. Rudolph C, Rudolph A, Hostetter M, Lister G, Siegel N: Rudolph's Pediatrics, 21st edition, New York, McGraw-Hill, 2002.

2. Behrman R, Kliegman R, Jenson H: Nelson's Textbook of Pediatrics, 17th edition, Philadelphia, W.B. Saunders, 2003.

3. McMillan J, deAngelis C, Feigin R, Warshaw J: Oski's Pediatrics—Principles and Practice, 3rd edition, Philadelphia, Lippincott, Williams & Wilkins, 1999.

4. Shah B, Laude T: Atlas of Pediatric Clinical Diagnosis, 1st edition, Philadelphia, W.B. Saunders, 2000.

5. Jones K: Smith's Recognizable Patterns of Human Malformation, 5th edition, Philadelphia, W.B. Saunders, 1997.

GYNECOLOGY

Amenorrhea

PRIMARY AMENORRHEA

Definitions
1. Absence of menstruation by the age of 16 with normal breast and pubic hair development
2. Lack of menses by the age of 14 years without normal breast/pubic hair development
3. No menses within 2 years by SMR stage 4

Etiology
- Hypothalamic/pituitary
- Hypothyroidism
- Gonadal
- Hormone defect

Initial Labs
- Karyotype
- CBC
- ESR
- Thyroid studies
- Hormone levels:
    - Prolactin
    - FSH
    - LH

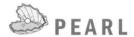

PEARL

Must consider **Turner syndrome** in girls with pubertal delay, short stature and amenorrhea

SECONDARY AMENORRHEA

Definition
- Cessation of menstruation for 6 months AFTER regular menses for more than 3 consecutive months

Etiology
- **Pregnancy** (most common)
- Anovulatory cycles (after first 2 years of menarche)

Vulvovaginitis

Etiology

INFECTIONS

- Candidiasis
- Group A and B beta-hemolytic streptococci
- Pinworms (*Enterobius vermicularis*)
- *S. aureus*
- STD

NONSPECIFIC (70% OF CASES)

- **Fecal contamination**
- Foreign body
- Chemical irritation
- Tight clothing
- Labial adhesions

Manifestations

- **Vaginal discharge** (most common)
    - —Green/brown
    - —pH: 4.7–6.5
    - —Fetid odor
- Erythema
- Irritation
- Dysuria
- Pruritus

Labs

URINE

- Epithelial cells
- Occasional WBCs

Treatment

- Sitz baths
- Proper hygiene
- Recurrent vulvovaginitis—treat with antibiotics

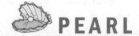

PEARL

Labial adhesions are treated with estrogen creams.

Vaginal Discharge Pearls

FOREIGN BODY

- **Brown, bloody** discharge
- Younger girls—typically toilet paper
- Older girls—retained tampon

PHYSIOLOGIC

- White, odorless mucoid discharge
- **Precedes menarche** by 3 to 6 months
- May continue for years following menarche
- pH—4.5
- Gram stain: **lactobacilli (rod-shaped)**
- Saline prep: epithelial cells

CANDIDA ALBICANS VAGINITIS

- Pruritus
- **"Cottage cheese"** or white curdy discharge
- KOH prep: budding yeast and hyphae
- Treated with imidazole cream
- Associated with diabetes mellitus and systemic antibiotic use

RHABDOMYOSARCOMA

- **Grapelike mass protruding through vagina**
- Treatment: resection
- Prognosis good if resectable; poor if not

Vaginal Bleeding

Etiology

- Pregnancy/abortion/ectoptic pregnancy
- **Foreign body** (tampon or IUD)
- Sexually transmitted disease
- Thyroid disease
- Blood dyscrasia (**von Willebrand disease**)
    - —Associated with very heavy menses
- **Dysfunctional uterine bleeding**
    - —Irregular/painless/prolonged endometrial bleeding
    - —> 10 days of bleeding
    - —Usually due to anovulatory cycles in adolescents
    - —Can occur for 1 to 2 years

Treatment

- Depends on level of anemia/hemodynamic status

NORMAL HEMATOCRIT (HCT)
- Reassurance and monitoring

MILD ANEMIA (HCT > 9 MG/DL)
- Ferrous sulfate
- Estrogen/progesterone or progesterone alone

SEVERE ANEMIA (HCT < 8 MG/DL) OR HEMODYNAMIC INSTABILITY
- Hospitalization for stabilization
- Intravenous conjugated estrogen
- Blood transfusion may be indicated

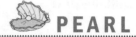

PEARL

Do not want to give *oral* estrogen as sole agent.

Abnormal Puberty

Precocious Puberty

- Appearance of puberty before age 8 years in a female
- Appearance of puberty before 9 years in a male

Initial Management

- Perform a **bone age** radiograph

Types

TRUE OR CENTRAL PRECOCIOUS PUBERTY
- Due to early maturation of the hypothalamic secretion of GnRH (**GnRH-dependent**)
- **Bone age: advanced**
- Differential diagnosis:
  - CNS disorders (tumors)
  - Idiopathic

"PSEUDOCOMPLETE" PRECOCIOUS PUBERTY
- **GnRH independent**
- **Bone age: advanced**
- Differential diagnosis:
  - Gonadotropin-secreting tumors (teratomas)
  - Gonadal tumors
  - Adrenal tumors
  - Iatrogenic or exogenous exposure to estrogen containing drugs
  - McCune-Albright syndrome

HYPOTHYROIDISM
- **Bone age: delayed**

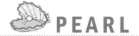

PEARL

In females involves *both* breast and pubic hair development, and in males involves *both* pubic hair and genital development.

Premature Thelarche

Definition

- Isolated breast development in girls before 8 years of age
- Usually occurs between 1 to 4 years old
- Variation of normal pubertal development
- No pubic hair development/linear growth acceleration

Etiology

TRANSIENT ELEVATION OF ESTROGEN FROM:

- Functional ovarian cyst (rule out via ultrasound)
- Fluctuations in pituitary gonadotropin secretion
- Medications—estrogen cream/oral contraceptives

Follow-up

- Must evaluate every 6 to 12 months for precocious puberty

Prognosis

- Spontaneous regression of breast enlargement

REFERENCES

1. Rudolph C, Rudolph A, Hostetter M, Lister G, Siegel N: Rudolph's Pediatrics, 21st edition, New York, McGraw-Hill, 2002.

2. Behrman R, Kliegman R, Jenson H: Nelson's Textbook of Pediatrics, 17th edition, Philadelphia, W.B. Saunders, 2003.

3. McMillan J, deAngelis C, Feigin R, Warshaw J: Oski's Pediatrics—Principles and Practice, 3rd edition, Philadelphia, Lippincott, Williams & Wilkins, 1999.

HEMATOLOGY

Autoimmune Hemolytic Anemia

Etiology

- Postinfectious (mycoplasma, Epstein-Barr virus)
- Systemic lupus erythematosus
- Drugs (penicillin)
- Malignancy (non-Hodgkin's lymphoma)

Manifestations

- Acute onset
- Fatigue
- Dizziness
- Splenomegaly
- Pallor
- Jaundice
- Dark-urine

Labs

- Anemia (normochromic/normocytic)
- Positive direct/indirect coombs
- Reticulocytosis
- Smear with microspherocytosis
- High bilirubin
- Antibodies
    IgG—(**warm**—SLE, lymphomas)
    IgM—(**cold**—mycoplasma, EBV)
    IgG—(**cold**—"Donath Landsteiner"—syphilis)

Treatment

- Supportive care
- Corticosteroids
- IVIG
- Splenectomy
- Immunosuppressive agents
- Transfusion of PRBC

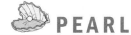 **PEARL**

Watch for anemia with **reticulocytosis** with positive Coombs' test.

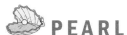 **PEARL**

Transfused PRBCs likely will be hemolyzed.

Sickle Cell Disease

Manifestations

DACTYLITIS
- Classic presenting manifestation
- Symmetric **swollen hands/feet**
- Occurs after 6 months of age

VASO-OCCLUSIVE CRISES
- Bone infarction
- Pain/swelling

APLASTIC CRISES
- Associated with **parvovirus B19**
- Severe anemia with **no reticulocytosis**
- Treat with transfusion

ACUTE CHEST SYNDROME
- Fever, chest pain and respiratory complaints
- Life-threatening
- Treat with simple/exchange transfusion

STROKE
- Focal neurologic signs
- Treat with simple/exchange transfusions
- Transfuse first then image via MRI/CT
- Requires **chronic transfusion therapy**

SPLENIC SEQUESTRATION
- Occurs commonly from 6 months to 3 years old
- Functional asplenia in early childhood
- Rapid increase in spleen size
- Life-threatening
- Treat with transfusion

FUNCTIONAL ASPLENIA
- At risk for sepsis/death from **encapsulated organisms**
- Require pneumovax

OSTEOMYELITIS
- *Salmonella* osteomyelitis

Sickle Cell Disease *continued*

Inheritance

■ Autosomal recessive

Labs

■ Anemia (sickling RBCs on smear)
■ Reticulocytosis
■ Hyperbilirubinemia
■ **Howell-Jolly bodies**

Diagnosis

■ Hemoglobin electrophoresis (**Hb S**)

Treatment

■ Pain management
■ Folic acid
■ Hydration
■ Hydroxyurea (stimulates **Hb F**)
■ Prophylactic penicillin
■ Pneumovax vaccine
■ Transfusion

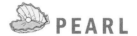 **PEARL**

Howell-Jolly bodies are spherical granules seen in RBCs due to asplenia.

Glucose-6-Phosphate Dehydrogenase (G6PD) Deficiency

Inheritance

■ X-linked

Pathophysiology

Hemolysis following exposure to oxidant stress:
■ Naphthalene (mothballs)
■ Infections (viral/bacterial)
■ Primaquine
■ Sulfonamides
■ Fava beans

Manifestations

■ Splenomegaly
■ Unconjugated hyperbilirubinemia
■ Anemia
■ Reticulocytosis
■ **Heinz bodies**

Diagnosis

■ Measure enzyme activity in the RBC

Treatment

■ Supportive
■ Transfusion (if severe anemia)

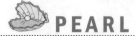

PEARL

Watch for anemia with reticulocytosis and negative direct/indirect Coombs' test.

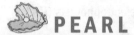

PEARL

Spherocytosis (autosomal dominant) will also present with anemia, reticulocytosis and negative Coombs' test but will have spherocytes with an **elevated MCHC**. Diagnose spherocytosis via *osmotic fragility test.*

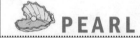

PEARL

Can get "false normal" G6PD enzyme level if check during a crisis because young RBCs have higher levels of G6PD enzyme. Must repeat after recovery.

Methemoglobinemia

Etiology

DRUGS

- Anesthetics
- Nitrites/nitrates
- Sulfa-based antibiotics
- Phenacetin

CONGENITAL

- Deficiency of NADPH-dependent methemoglobin reductase

Manifestations

- **Cyanosis**
- Hypoxia

Diagnosis

- Co-oximetry studies
- Pulse oximeter will read **falsely high**

Treatment

- Methylene blue

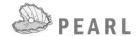

PEARL

Occurs in infants who live in rural areas (i.e., farms) who ingest nitrate contaminated well-water.

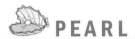

PEARL

Chocolate-dark arterial blood that does not turn red when exposed to air may be described in question.

Von Willebrand's Disease

Inheritance

- Usually autosomal dominant
- Most common hereditary bleeding disorder

Pathogenesis

- Defect in the production of von Willebrand protein

Features

- Epistaxis
- Ecchymoses
- Menorrhagia
- Postoperative bleeding

Labs

- **Bleeding time: prolonged**
- **PTT: prolonged**
- PT: normal
- Platelets: normal

Diagnosis

- Decreased VwF activity (ristocetin)

Treatment

- Desmopressin acetate
- VwF concentrate
- Aminocaproic acid (for minor mucosal bleeding)

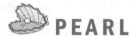

PEARL

May describe an adolescent female with excessive bleeding with menses or child with prolonged bleeding after tooth removal.

Hemophilias

HEMOPHILIA A

- Deficiency of factor VIII
- X-linked
- **Intracranial hemorrhage, joint bleeding and muscle bleeds**
- Diagnose: decreased factor VIII activity

Labs

- Bleeding time: normal
- **PTT: prolonged**
- PT: normal
- Platelets: normal
  - VwF assay: normal

Treatment

- Factor VIII concentrate and DDAVP

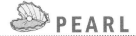

PEARL

Typically presents as toddlers with increased bruising following minor trauma.

HEMOPHILIA B

- Deficiency of factor IX
- X-linked
- **Intracranial hemorrhage, joint bleeding and muscle bleeds**
- Diagnose: decreased factor IX activity

Labs

- Bleeding time: normal
- **PTT: prolonged**
- PT: normal
- Platelets: normal
- VwF assay: normal

Treatment

- Factor IX concentrate

Hemorrhagic Disease of the Newborn

CLASSIC FORM (MOST COMMON)

- Occurs in **breast-fed** infants who **did not receive vitamin K** prophylaxis (i.e., baby born at home)
- Occurs second to seventh day of life
- Presents with bleeding after circumcision, melena, intracranial hemorrhage
- Prolonged PT and PTT
- Treatment: IV/IM vitamin K

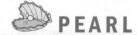

PEARL

Rarely occurs in formula-fed infants because formula has vitamin K.

EARLY FORM

- Occurs in the first 24 hours and is linked to **maternal medications** that interfere with vitamin K storage.
  - Warfarin
  - Anticonvulsants (phenobarbital, phenytoin)
  - Rifampin
  - Isoniazid
- Presents with bleeding, melena, intracranial hemorrhage, cephalohematoma
- Prolonged PT and PTT
- Treatment: IV/IM vitamin K

LATE FORM

- Occurs at 2 to 8 weeks of age secondary to decreased supply of vitamin K from diarrhea, **cystic fibrosis, hepatitis or celiac disease**
- Presents with bleeding, melena, intracranial hemorrhage
- Prolonged PT and PTT
- Treatment: IV/IM vitamin K

Differential Diagnosis for Macrocytic Anemia

FOLATE DEFICIENCY

- **Hypersegmentation of neutrophils**
- Dietary deficiency—no green vegetables or fruit
- No neurologic findings
- Diagnosed by low concentration of folate in red blood cells
- Must check B_{12} in all patients suspected of folate deficiency to avoid a misdiagnosis and potential neurologic complications
- Treatment: folic acid

B_{12} DEFICIENCY

Etiology

- Dietary deficiency occurs in, or in infants breast-fed by, **strict vegans**
- Following small bowel resection—**terminal ileum**
- Bacterial overgrowth
- Pernicious anemia (loss of intrinsic factor gastric parietal cells)
  - —Associated with polyendocrinopathy syndrome

Manifestations

- Glossitis
- Neuropathy (subacute combined degeneration of the spinal cord)
  - —Loss of vibrational/positional sense
  - —Depression/dementia
  - —Ataxia

Labs

- **Hypersegmentation of neutrophils**

Diagnosis

- Low serum B_{12}
- Schilling test

Treatment

- Vitamin B_{12}

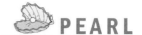

PEARL

Occurs in children fed **goat's milk or powdered milk.**

Microcytic Anemias

IRON DEFICIENCY

- **Very common**
- Occurs between 6 months and 24 months
- Associated with **diet high in cow's milk** or low-iron formula
- Manifestations include palor, fatigue and pica
- Labs
  - MCV: low
  - RDW: **high**
  - Free erythrocyte protoporphyrin: **high**
  - TIBC: **high**
  - Ferritin: **low**
  - Iron: **low**
- Treatment: iron 3 to 6 mg/kg/day
- Reticulocyte count should increase in *3 to 5 days*

LEAD POISONING

- CDC definition: lead $> 10\mu g/dL$
- Usually secondary to **lead-containing paint** in homes built before 1950
- Manifestations include pica, abdominal colic, neuropathy, constipation, developmental delay and attention disorders
- Labs
  - MCV: low
  - RDW: **high**
  - Free erythrocyte protoporphyrin: **high**
  - TIBC: normal
  - Ferritin: normal
  - Iron: normal
- Treatment: environmental clean-up and dimercaprol (BAL), edetate calcium-disodium (EDTA) or oral succimer (DMSA)

THALASSEMIA

- **α-Thalassemias result from reduced synthesis of α-globin chains**
  - associated with Asian or African background
- **Types of α-Thalassemias:**
  - Major (4 genes deleted)—death in utero
  - H Disease (3 genes deleted)—severe anemia
  - Minor (2 genes deleted)—mild anemia
  - Silent (1 gene deleted)—asymptomatic

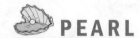 **PEARL**

Also occurs with adolescent females secondary to iron loss with menses.

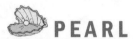 **PEARL**

Iron-deficiency anemia is associated with a high RDW, whereas the thalassemias are not.

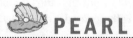 **PEARL**

RBC smear may demonstrate basophilic stippling.

Microcytic Anemias *continued*

- Labs
  - MCV: normal
  - RDW: normal
  - Free erythrocyte protoporphyrin: normal
  - TIBC: normal
  - Ferritin: normal
  - Iron: normal
- Treatment
  - α-Thalassemia minor not treated
  - H disease treated with folic acid; may need transfusions

β-THALASSEMIA

- **β-Thalassemias result from reduced synthesis of β-globin chains**
  - Associated with Mediterranean background
- **Types of β-Thalassemias**
  - Major (homozygous)—severe anemia, **hepatosplenomegaly** and bone marrow hyperplasia with **frontal bossing**
  - Minor (heterozygous)—mild anemia
- Labs
  - MCV: normal
  - RDW: normal
  - Free erythrocyte protoporphyrin: normal
  - TIBC: normal
  - Ferritin: normal
  - Iron: normal
  - **Hemoglobin A$_2$**: elevated
- Treatment
  - Minor—monitored
  - Major—chronic transfusions

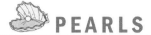

PEARLS

Transient erythroblastopenia of childhood occurs between 6 months and 3 years of age and is self-limited (most children recover in 1 to 2 months). Lab analysis finds normal adenosine deaminase activity and hemoglobin F.

In **Diamond-Blackfan syndrome**, the anemia develops between 2 to 6 months and is associated with an elevated adenosine deaminase activity, hemoglobin F. Treatment is corticosteroids and/or chronic infusions.

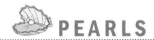

PEARLS

Skull radiograph will demonstrate the "hair-like" appearance due to the vertical trabeculae.

Iron overload develops in all patients with β-thalassemia major and accumulates in liver, heart, pancreas ("**bronzed diabetes**") and skin, and patients must be chelated. Myocardial siderosis is a major factor in death.

Acute Idiopathic Thrombocytopenia Purpura

Etiology

- Usually preceded by viral infection by 1 to 4 weeks

Epidemiology

- 1 to 4 years of age

Manifestations

- Acute onset
- **Patients appear well**
- Petechiae/purpura
- Bruising
- Bleeding

Labs

- Decreased platelets
- Large platelets
- **Abnormal bleeding time**
- Normal PT and PTT

Complications

- Intracranial hemorrhage (platelets < 20,000)

Treatment

- If platelets > 30,000: monitor CBC closely
- IVIG
- Prednisone
- Anti-D therapy (given to Rh-positive individuals)

Prognosis

- Excellent; usually self-limited (90%)

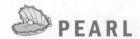

PEARL

If describe thrombocytopenia in question and show radiograph of arm must consider TAR (thrombocytopenia-absent radius syndrome).

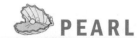

PEARL

Prednisone usually not given without performing a bone marrow aspirate to avoid masking a leukemia.

REFERENCES

1. Beutler E, Lichtman M, Coller B, Kipps T, Seligsohn U: Williams Hematology, 6th edition, New York, McGraw-Hill, 2001.

2. Behrman R, Kliegman R, Jenson H: Nelson Textbook of Pediatrics, 17th edition, Philadelphia, W.B. Saunders, 2003.

3. McMillan J, DeAngelis C, Feigin R, Warshaw J: Oski's Pediatrics—Principles and Practice, 3rd edition, Philadelphia, Lippincott, Williams & Wilkins, 1999.

4. Rudolph C, Rudolph A, Hostetter M, Lister G, Siegel N: Rudolph's Pediatrics, 21st edition, New York, McGraw-Hill, 2002.

IMMUNOLOGY

B-Cell Immunodeficiencies

TRANSIENT HYPOGAMMAGLOBULINEMIA

- Normal B- and T-cell populations
- **Antibodies to blood antigens** and appropriate titers following immunization
- Treatment: antibiotics for infections but usually do not require IVIG
- Resolves by 18 to 36 months

X-LINKED AGAMMAGLOBULINEMIA

- Males only
- Healthy until *6 to 9 months* of age
- **Pyogenic bacterial infections** (OM, pneumonia, meningitis)
  - *S. pneumoniae*
  - *H. influenzae*
- Susceptible to **enteroviral infections**
- Hypoplasia of tonsils, adenoids and lymph nodes
- No circulating B cells
- IgG, IgA, IgM and IgE are decreased or absent
- **No antibodies to blood groups** and no antibody titer rise following immunization
- Do not give live virus vaccinations
- Treatment: **IVIG**

IgA DEFICIENCY

- Most common immunodeficiency
- Bacterial sinusitis and pneumonias
- Increased incidence of celiac, autoimmune diseases and malignancies
- Do not treat with IVIG
- Treatment: antibiotics for infections

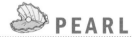 **PEARL**

Must receive **washed blood products** owing to increased risk of anaphylaxis due to IgA antibodies.

COMMON VARIABLE IMMUNODEFICIENCY

- Typically presents 15 to 35 years of age
- Increased **pyogenic infections** (especially sinus disease)
- Increased autoimmune diseases (SLE, arthritis) and malignancies

B-Cell Immunodeficiencies *continued*

- "Sprue-like" syndrome with diarrhea, malabsorption and steatorrhea
- Noncaseating granulomas of lungs, spleen, liver and skin
- Anemias
- Labs: decreased total immunoglobulins, decreased IgG
- Treatment: IVIG

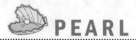

PEARL

IgA and IgM may vary from normal to absent.

T-Cell Immunodeficiencies

DIGEORGE SYNDROME

- Microdeletion from chromosome 22q11.2
- Dysmorphogenesis of third and fourth pharyngeal pouches
- Hypoplasia of thymus and parathyroid glands
- Abnormal facies ("fish-shaped" mouth, small jaw)
- **Hypocalcemic seizures** (most common presentation)
- Conotruncal cardiac disorders
- Normal B cells with variable antibody levels/function
- Usually lymphopenia (< 1500)
- Infections from **opportunistic infections:**
  –Fungi
  –Viruses
  –*Pneumocystis carinii*
- Treatment: prophylactic antibiotics, thymic tissue transplant and BMT

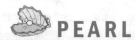

PEARL

Chest radiograph will *not* have a thymic shadow.

HYPER IGM

- Predominantly X-linked
- Low IgG and IgA **with markedly elevated IgM** (150–1000 mg/dl)
- B cells cannot undergo isotype switching
- Lymphadenopathy
- Symptomatic during first year of life with **pyogenic infections:**
  - Recurrent otitis media
  - sinusitis
  - pneumonia (**P. carinii common initial infection**)
  - tonsillitis
- Associated with sclerosing cholangitis, liver disease and hepatoma
- Treatment: IVIG

Combined T- and B-Cell Immunodeficiencies

SEVERE COMBINED IMMUNODEFICIENCY DISEASE

- X-linked, autosomal recessive and sporadic
- Presents in **first 3 months of life** with failure to thrive, diarrhea, thrush and respiratory infections
- Infections from **viruses (CMV), bacteria, fungi *(Candida)*, and protozoa *(P. carinii)***
- No thymus
- Lymphopenia (< 1500 cells/μL)
- Hypogammaglobulinemia with no antibody production following immunization
- Usually paucity of B cells
- Prognosis: death in first year of life
- Treatment: BMT

Syndromes with Immunodeficiency

WISKOTT-ALDRICH

- X-linked recessive
- Triad of:
  - **Eczema**
  - **Thrombocytopenia (small defective platelets)**
  - **Infections**
- Cellular and humoral immunity defects
- Often present with prolonged bleeding from circumcision/bloody diarrhea
- Susceptible to **capsular bacterial organisms,** including *Pneumococcus, Meningococcus* and *H. influenzae*
- Prognosis: death in adolescence
- Treatment: BMT

ATAXIA TELANGIECTASIA

- Autosomal recessive
- Progressive cerebellar ataxia—starts after initiation of walking
- Oculocutaneous telangiectasias—begins at age 3 years
- Chronic sinopulmonary disease
- Varying degrees of T- and B-cell abnormalities
- 40% of patients have IgA deficiency
- Sensitive to ionizing radiation for lymphoreticular malignancies
- Increased risk of malignancies

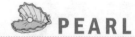

PEARL

Classic board question shows an eye with telangiectasia.

Phagocytic Dysfunction Diseases

CHRONIC GRANULOMATOUS DISEASE

- X-linked (65%) and AR (35%)
- Infections with **catalase-positive organisms**— *S. aureus, S. epidermidis, Serratia marcescens, Salmonella and E. coli*
- Also at risk for infections with Aspergillus
- Presents < 2 years old with draining lymphadenitis, hepatosplenomegaly, pneumonia, osteomyelitis and abscesses.
- Diagnosis: **NBT (cannot reduce NBT dye)**
- Treatment: Prophylactic antibiotics, IFNγ

CHEDIAK-HIGASHI SYNDROME

- Autosomal recessive
- Infections from a variety of bacterial organisms
- Multisystem findings include **partial albinism,** central nervous system abnormalities and "silvery hair"
- Large **granules in neutrophils and eosinophils**
- Increased risk of lymphoreticular cancers
- Poor prognosis without bone marrow transplant

HYPER IGE SYNDROME (JOB'S SYNDROME)

- **"Cold abscesses"**—no redness, heat or pain
- Recurrent *Staphyloccus* **infections** of skin, subcutaneous tissues, lungs, upper airways and bones.
- Coarse facies
- Increased IgE (>2000 IU/ml)
- Blood and tissue eosinophilia
- Treatment: prophylactic antibiotics

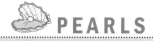 **PEARLS**

May show chest radiograph with pneumatoceles.

LEUKOCYTE ADHESION DEFECT TYPE 1 (LAD)

- Autosomal recessive
- Delayed umbilical cord detachment (> than 3 weeks)
- Recurrent **pyogenic infections** from *S. aureus, Pseudomonas* and *Klebsiella*
- Periodontal disease
- **Increased peripheral neutrophil count**
- Treatment: BMT and prophylactic antibiotics

Complement Disorders

C1 INHIBITOR DEFICIENCY

■ Develop **hereditary angioedema**

TERMINAL COMPLEMENT COMPONENT DEFICIENCIES

■ Increased risk of *Neisseria* **infections**

C3, C2, C4, C1Q, C1R AND C1S DEFICIENCIES

■ Increased risk of **discoid lupus, SLE,** vasculitis and glomerulonephritis

HIV

Transmission

80% OF PEDIATRIC CASES DUE TO MATERNAL TRANSMISSION

- 25% if HIV-infected mother not treated
- 8% if HIV-infected mother treated with AZT (no breast-feeding)

Diagnosis

INFANTS YOUNGER THAN 18 MONTHS

- Two positive cultures of HIV (gold standard)
- Two positive DNA PCR

CHILDREN OLDER THAN 18 MONTHS

- Two positive ELISA tests and western blot

Immunizations

FOLLOW AAP GUIDELINES EXCEPT:

- No oral polio

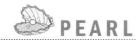

PEARL

HIV-infected mothers should be advised **not to breast-feed** if safe-alternative formulas are available.

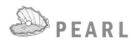

PEARL

HIV-infected children may have elevated immunoglobulins.

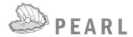

PEARL

HIV-positive patients can receive the **MMR vaccine**.

Poison Ivy Exposure

Pathophysiology
- Type IV hypersensitivity reaction

Rash
- Pruritic macules leading to papules, vesicles and bullae
- Rash can spread for several days following exposure
- Exposure to fluid does not spread rash

Treatment
- Oral steroids (10- to 14-day course)
- Antihistamines
- Untreated; the rash can last 2 to 4 weeks

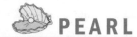

PEARL

Lesions form **linear and angulated** patterns that correspond to sites of exposure.

REFERENCES

1. Parslow T, Stites D, Terr A, Imboden J: Medical Immunology, 10th edition, New York, Lange Medical Books, 2001.

2. Behrman R, Kliegman R, Jenson H: Nelson Textbook of Pediatrics, 17th edition, Philadelphia, W.B. Saunders, 2003.

3. McMillan J, DeAngelis C, Feigin R, Warshaw J: Oski's Pediatrics—Principles and Practice, 3rd edition, Philadelphia, Lippincott, Williams & Wilkins, 1999.

4. Rudolph C, Rudolph A, Hostetter M, Lister G, Siegel N: Rudolph's Pediatrics, 21st edition, New York, McGraw-Hill, 2002.

INFECTIOUS DISEASE

Diarrhea

SHIGELLA

- Gram-negative bacilli
- Watery/bloody diarrhea, fever, and abdominal pain
- CBC with **increased bands**
- Usually **treated** with antibiotics (ampicillin, trimethoprim-methoxazole)
- Excluded from day care until symptoms have resolved and stool cultures are negative

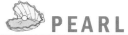 **PEARL**

Associated with Reiter syndrome, hemolytic-uremic syndrome and new-onset **seizures**.

SALMONELLA

- Gram-negative bacilli
- Watery/bloody diarrhea, fever, and abdominal pain
- Healthy children with nontyphoid *Salmonella* are **not treated**
- Treatment does not shorten duration and can prolong excretion
- Antibiotics (ampicillin, trimethoprim-methoxazole) indicated for:
  - Infants < 3 months
  - Typhoid fever
  - Invasive disease (osteomyelitis or meningitis)
  - Immunosuppressed patients/HIV
  - Hemoglobinopathies
  - Malignant neoplasms

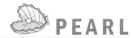 **PEARL**

Can be transmitted via infected pets, including turtles and/or iguanas.

E. coli Diarrhea

ENTEROHEMORRHAGIC E.COLI O157:H7 (EHEC)

- Usually begins as nonbloody diarrhea and progresses to grossly bloody
- Found in hamburger and unpasteurized milk/apple cider
- Associated with the development of **hemolytic-uremia syndrome (HUS)**
- Risks of developing HUS:
  - Extremes of age
  - Bloody diarrhea
  - Fever
  - Leukocytosis
  - Female gender
  - Mental retardation
- Not treated with antibiotics

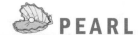 **PEARL**

Treatment with antibiotics during the infection may increase the likelihood of the patient developing HUS.

ENTEROTOXIGENIC E.COLI (ETEC)

- Usually nonbloody diarrhea
- **"Travelers diarrhea"**
- Not treated with antibiotics
- Self-limited

ENTEROPATHOGENIC E.COLI (EPEC)

- Usually nonbloody diarrhea
- Causes acute/chronic diarrhea in neonates and young children
- Found in developing countries with poor sanitary conditions
- Not treated with antibiotics
- Uncommon in USA

ENTEROINVASIVE E.COLI (EIEC)

- Usually *bloody* diarrhea with fever
- Dysentery similar to *Shigella*
- Contaminated foods are source
- Not treated with antibiotics

Urinary Tract Infection/Pyelonephritis

Etiology

- *E. coli* (most common)
- *Klebsiella*
- *Proteus*
- *Pseudomonas*

Manifestations

- Vomiting
- Fever
- Flank pain
- Abdominal pain
- Pain with urination
- Urgency/frequency

Diagnosis

SUPRAPUBIC PUNCTURE URINALYSIS
- Few gram-negative organisms
- >1,000 cfu/ml of bacterial organisms

BLADDER CATHETERIZATION URINALYSIS
- 10,000 cfu/ml of bacterial organisms

CLEAN-CATCH (MIDSTREAM) URINALYSIS
- >100,000 cfu/ml of bacterial organisms

Treatment

- Initially IV antibiotics (i.e., cefotaxime)
- Change to PO antibiotics after vomiting/fever cease
- Treat for 10–14 days

Work-up

- Ultrasound
- VCUG
  - Girls < 5 years old after first UTI
  - All boys
  - Patients with pyelonephritis (febrile UTI)
  - Girls > 5 years old after second UTI

Bronchiolitis

Etiology
- Respiratory syncytial virus (most common)
- Parainfluenza virus
- Adenovirus

Epidemiology
- Occurs in children aged 3 months to 2 years

Manifestations
- Rhinorrhea
- Cough
- Tachypnea
- Wheezing
- Dyspnea
- Fever

Management
- Supportive
- Oxygen
- Frequent suctioning
- Nebulized albuterol/epinephrine may be beneficial

Fifth Disease

Etiology

- Human parvovirus B19

Manifestations

SKIN

- **"Slapped cheek" facial rash**
- Lacy, reticular rash on trunk and extremities
- Rash preceded 7 to 10 days by fever, headache and myalgias
- Rash worsened by sunlight, heat, exercise and stress

Complications

JOINTS

- Arthritis
  - Symmetric
  - Polyarticular: hands, wrist and knees
- Usually occurs in adolescents
- Self-limited; resolves in 2 to 4 weeks

HEMATOLOGIC

- Transient aplastic crisis
- **No reticulocytosis**
- Occurs in chronic hemolytic diseases
  - Sickle cell disease/thalassemia
  - Hereditary spherocytosis
  - Pyruvate kinase deficiency

FETUS

- Primary maternal infection associated with nonimmune fetal hydrops/fetal demise
- Viral-induced red cell aplasia
- May need intrauterine blood transfusions

Diagnosis

- Clinically; IgM for parvovirus B19

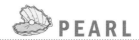 **PEARL**

Blood transfusion may be necessary if hemodynamically unstable.

Roseola (Erythema Subitum)

Etiology
- Human herpes virus 6

Manifestations
EXANTHUM SUBITUM
- Children < 3 years old
- High fever (101–106 °F)
- Fever persists for 3 to 5 days
- Fever usually **abruptly resolves**, and pink/red papules appear on trunk and spread to extremities, neck and face

Diagnosis
- Clinically

Treatment
- Supportive

Tuberculosis

Etiology

- *M. tuberculosis* (acid-fast bacillus)

Transmission

- Air-borne mucous droplet

Manifestations

- Cough
- Weight loss
- Night sweats/fevers
- Meningitis
- Bone lesions
- Renal

Radiographic Findings

CHEST X-RAY

- Lymphadenopathy of the hilar, mediastinal, or cervical nodes; atelectasis, infiltrate, cavitary lesion or pleural effusion

Diagnosis

- Culture (sputum, pleural fluid, CSF or gastric aspirates)
- Biopsy

Treatment

LATENT (POSITIVE SKIN TEST/NO DISEASE)

- 9 months of isoniazid

PULMONARY

- 2 months of isoniazid/rifampin/pyrazinamide, followed by 4 months of isoniazid/rifampin

Affected Health Care Workers

RETURN TO WORK AFTER

1. Receiving antituberculous therapy
2. Cough has resolved
3. Three consecutive negative sputum smears for acid-fast bacillus

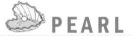

PEARL

Best specimen is an early morning gastric aspirate.

Tuberculin Skin Test

Significance

■ A positive tuberculin skin test indicates a **likely infection**.

Definition of Positive Test

INDURATION > 15 MM

■ Children > 4 years old; no risk factors

INDURATION > 10 MM

■ Children with increased exposure to TB
- Travel to areas where TB endemic
- Born in, or parents from, area where TB endemic
- Exposed to adults with HIV, homeless, users of illicit drugs, migrant farm workers, incarcerated or residents of nursing homes
■ Children at risk of disseminated disease
- < 4 years of age
- Systemic illness, including renal failure, malnutrition, diabetes mellitus lymphoma or Hodgkin's disease

INDURATION > 5 MM

■ Children in close contact with known/suspected case of TB
■ Children suspected to have TB
- Positive chest radiograph
- TB in differential diagnosis of illness

Infectious Mononucleosis

Etiology

- Epstein-Barr virus

Epidemiology

- Transmitted via oropharyngeal secretions; "kissing disease"
- Incubation: 30 to 50 days

Manifestations

- Fever
- Exudative pharyngitis/tonsillar hypertrophy
- Lymphadenopathy
- Hepatosplenomegaly

Labs

- Leukocytosis (**atypical lymphocytes**)

Diagnosis

- Serology
- Monospot (50% negative if < 4 years old)

Complications

- Splenic rupture
- Hemolytic anemia/thrombocytopenia
- Meningitis/seizures
- Guillain-Barré syndrome

Treatment

- Corticosteroids for life-threatening complications:
    - —Airway obstruction
    - —Hemolytic anemia
    - —Thrombocytopenia
    - —Meningitis
- Avoid contact sports until spleen size normalizes.

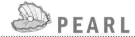

PEARL

Morbilliform rash after penicillin is not an IgE allergic reaction.

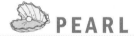

PEARL

30% incidence of coexistent group A beta-hemolytic streptococcal infection.

Herpes Simplex Virus (HSV)

ENCEPHALITIS

- Presentation: fever, mental status changes and focal seizures
- EEG with PLEDS (periodic lateralized epileptiform discharges) in temporal lobes
- MRI: **increased temporal lobe signal**
- CSF: **RBCs** with elevated lymphocytes
- Diagnosis: PCR of CSF for HSV
- Treatment: IV acyclovir

ACUTE STOMATITIS

- Presentation: fever, pain in mouth, refusal to drink/eat and oral lesions
- Self-limited
- May need to initiate IV hydration if poor PO intake
- Treatment: PO acyclovir
- Acyclovir should be started within 3 days of symptoms

ECZEMA HERPETICUM

- Infection of **eczematous skin with herpes virus**
- Vesicles form over eczema
- Wide denudation of skin can occur
- Can be mild to *life-threatening*
- At risk for secondary infections, large fluid losses and electrolyte imbalances
- Treatment: IV or PO acyclovir
- Acyclovir should be started within 3 days of symptoms

Hepatitis

HEPATITIS A

- Fever, malaise, jaundice and anorexia
- Usually asymptomatic in children < 6 years old and symptomatic in others
- Transmitted via fecal-oral route
- Self-limited
- Can occur in **epidemics in child care facilities,** via food-borne or water-borne sources

HEPATITIS B

- Clinical symptoms can vary from asymptomatic to fulminant fatal hepatitis
- Transmitted via blood or body fluids
- Positive **HbsAg** indicates acute or chronically infected patient (first serologic marker to appear)
- **HbeAg** occurs during the acute phase and indicates a **highly infectious state**
- High risk for *fulminant hepatitis*
- No treatment is successful in majority of patients
- Chronic infection is associated with hepatocellular carcinoma

HEPATITIS C

- Fever, malaise, jaundice and anorexia
- High risk to develop *chronic infection*
- 70% develop chronic hepatitis and cirrhosis develops in 10% of these patients
- Cirrhosis can lead to hepatocellular carcinoma
- Hepatitis C is the leading reason for liver transplantation in the USA
- Treatment with **interferon-alpha**

Rocky Mountain Spotted Fever

Etiology

- *Rickettsia rickettsii* (vector—ticks)

Epidemiology

- Highest in the southeastern/mid-Atlantic states in spring
- Incubation: 2 to 12 days

Manifestations

- Fever
- Headache
- Arthralgias/myalgia
- Anorexia
- Photophobia
- Nausea/vomiting

Labs

- **Hyponatremia**
- **Thrombocytopenia**
- Leukopenia

Diagnosis

- Serologic antibody titers

Treatment

- Supportive
- Doxycycline, tetracycline or chloramphenicol

Complications

- DIC
- Cardiac failure/shock
- Death
- Neurologic

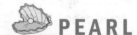 **PEARL**

Rash of macules/papules starts on **wrists/ankles** and spreads proximally to trunk/extremities. Usually becomes purpuric or petechial.

Miscellaneous Infections

INFECTION	TREATMENT	DIAGNOSTIC CLUES/COMMENTS
Listeria monocytogenes	Ampicillin	Unpasteurized dairy products Maternal infection is "flu-like"
Ascaris lumbricoides	Albendazole	Most prevalent worm infection
Chlamydia pneumoniae	Erythromycin	"Staccato cough" **Eosinophilia**
Entamoeba histolytica	Metronidazole	Bloody dysentery
Giardia lamblia	Metronidazole	Occurs in day-care centers Diarrhea
Bartonella henselae	Supportive	Cat scratch fever
Brucella	Doxycycline	Fever/arthritis/hepatosplenomegaly Unpasteurized dairy products
Tularemia	Gentamicin	Fever/headache/myalgias **Rabbit** is common source
Cryptococcosis	Amphotericin B	**Meningitis** Found in soil with bird dung
Coccidioidomycosis	Supportive	"Flu-like" syndrome **Desert travel** in Arizona/California
Pseuodmembranous colitis	Metronidazole	Diarrhea due to *C. difficile* toxin
Cryptosporidium	Supportive	Watery diarrhea Diagnose: oocysts in stool
H. pylori	Clarithromycin Metronidazole Omeprazole	Diagnose via: — Culture — Urease testing — Breath test (CO_2)
Yersinia pestis	Streptomycin	**Bubonic plague** Fever/lymphadenopathy Fleas on prairie dogs/squirrels Rural disease
Pasteurella multocida	Amox-clavulanate	Occurs with **cat bite**
S. aureus pneumonia	IV nafcillin	Develop **pneumatoceles**
Chlamydia psittaci	Tetracycline or erythromycin	Febrile respiratory infection **Birds** are reservoir
Histoplasmosis	Amphotericin B	**Bird dung along Mississippi River** Hepatosplenomegaly

Scabies

Etiology

- *Sarcoptes scabiei*

Transmission

- Via close contact with an individual/fomites (i.e., bedding)

Manifestations

INFANTS

- **Pruritic erythematous vesicles** or papules
- **Generalized**—covers face, trunk and extremities

OLDER CHILDREN AND ADULTS

- **Pruritic erythematous papules,** nodules or burrows
- Occurs on **interdigital webs,** flexor wrist, elbows, axillae folds, groin, breast and penis

Diagnosis

- Microscopic identification of mite (skin scrapping)

Treatment

- Permethrin cream 5% (first choice)
- Lindane 1%

Control Measures

- Treat all close contacts and family members.
- All clothing and bedding should be washed in hot water.

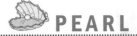

PEARL

Pruritic rash is a hypersensitivity reaction to mite and may persist for several weeks following treatment.

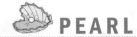

PEARL

Lindane causes neurotoxicity; avoid in infants, young children and pregnant/breast-feeding women.

Rabies

Animals Commonly Infected

- Bats, skunks, raccoons, foxes, coyotes, woodchucks, dogs, cats and ferrets

Postexposure Prophylaxis Indications

BATS, SKUNKS, RACCOONS, FOXES, COYOTES, WOODCHUCKS

- A bite or scratch
- Contamination of wound/scratch or mucous membrane with saliva
- **Any exposure to a bat** (i.e., in the same room as the patient)

DOGS, CATS AND FERRETS

- If observed animal (held for 10 days) shows signs of rabies
- Unknown/escaped dog (consult health officials)

Postexposure Prophylaxis

1. Washing of wound with soap and water
2. HRIG (human rabies immune globin) 50% should be locally infiltrated around the wound; should be given within *7 days* of starting the vaccine
3. HDVC (human diploid cell vaccine), RVA (rabies vaccine adsorbed) or PCEC (purified chick embryo cell culture) should be given IM on days 0, 3, 7, 14 and 28.

Prognosis

- Fatal encephalomyelitis without treatment

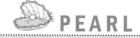 **PEARL**

Risk of rabies considered **low** from bites/scratches of rabbits, squirrels, guinea pigs, hamsters, mice or rats. Rarely need anti-rabies treatment.

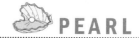 **PEARL**

Egg-allergic patients can obtain vaccine without skin testing.

Tetanus

Etiology
- *Clostridium tetani* (anaerobic gram-positive rod)
- Found in soil and human/animal feces

Pathophysiology
- *C. tetani* exotoxin causes severe generalized muscle spasms

Prophylaxis
History of 3 Previous Doses of Tetanus Toxoid

CLEAN—MINOR WOUNDS
- dT: Yes, if more than 10 years since last dose
- TIG: No

CONTAMINATED WOUNDS (DIRT/FECES/SALIVA/BURNS)
- dT: Yes, if more than 5 years since the last dose
- TIG: No

<3 Previous Doses of Tetanus Toxoid/Status Unknown

CLEAN—MINOR WOUNDS
- dT: Yes
- TIG: No

CONTAMINATED WOUNDS (DIRT/FECES/ SALIVA/ BURNS)
- dT: Yes
- TIG: Yes

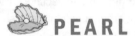

PEARL

For children younger than 7 years old, DTaP is recommended rather than dT.

Chemoprophylaxis

DIPHTHERIA

- All close contacts must receive treatment with erythromycin.
- Close contacts should receive a booster (diphtheria toxoid) if they have not had one in the past 5 years.
- Children who have had fewer than 3 doses of vaccine should begin active immunization.

INFLUENZA A

- Amantadine and rimantadine

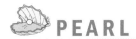

PEARL

Amantadine is associated with increased CNS side effects (i.e., seizures, behavior changes).

N. MENINGITIDIS

- Meningococcal vaccine for groups A, C, Y and W-135

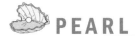

PEARL

The American College Health Association recommends immunization of college students with the meningococcal vaccine. Neither the AAP nor the CDC recommends the routine immunization.

RESPIRATORY SYNCYTIAL VIRUS

- RSV-IVIG and palivizumab (monoclonal antibody given IM)
- Used to prevent RSV in "at-risk" infants, including premature and children less than 2 years old with bronchopulmonary dysplasia

PERTUSSIS

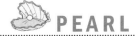

PEARL

RSV-IVIG increases complications and death if given to children with symptomatic cyanotic heart disease.

- All household contacts should be treated with erythromycin.
- Children less than 7 years who are unimmunized or who have had fewer than 4 doses of pertussis vaccine should also receive the pertussis-containing vaccine.
- Children who received their third dose $\geq$ 6 months ago should obtain the fourth dose.
- Children who received more than 4 doses of vaccine who are less than 7 years old and have not had a booster in the last 3 years should also receive a booster dose of DTaP.

Toxocariasis

Etiology

- Ingestion of dog/cat roundworm eggs (*T. canis* or *T. catti*)

Pathology

- Eggs hatch in gut
- Larvae migrate to any organ (visceral larva migrans)
- Eye involvement can occur (ocular larva migrans)

Manifestations

- Fever
- Cough
- Wheezing
- Urticaria
- Hepatomegaly

Diagnosis

- Liver biopsy
- Enzyme immunoassay

Treatment

- Usually resolves spontaneously
- Significant organ involvement—antihelminthics therapy

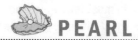

PEARL

Commonly occurs in children younger than 4 years old who engage in **pica** and are exposed to **dogs and cats**.

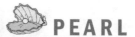

PEARL

Associated with significant **eosinophilia** and hypergammaglobulinemia.

Rubeola (Measles)

Manifestations

- **3 C's:**Coryza, cough and conjunctivitis
- **Koplik spots (pathognomonic)**—gray/white spots on buccal surface
- Maculopapular exanthem

Transmission

- Respiratory droplets

Diagnosis

- Antibody titers

Treatment

- Supportive
- Vitamin A (in developing countries)
- IVIG indications:
    - —Immunocompromised
    - —Pregnant
    - —Infant 6 to 12 months of age
    - —Infant less than 6 months (mother without immunity)

Complications

- **Pneumonia** (most common cause of death)
- Otitis media
- Encephalitis
- **Subacute sclerosing panencephalitis**
    - —Risk: 1 in 100,000 following natural infection
    - —Presentation:
        - Dementia
        - Myoclonus
        - Choreoathetosis
        - Extrapyramidal disorders
    - —Diagnosis: EEG pattern and antibodies in serum/CSF
    - —Prognosis: death (usually in 3 years)

Varicella

Lesions

■ Papules → vesicles → pustules → crusting
■ Erythema around a vesicle; "a dewdrop on a rose petal"

Epidemiology

■ Contagious: 1 to 2 days before to 5 days after lesions erupt
■ Incubation: 14 to 16 days
■ Isolate susceptible cases from day 8 to 21 following exposure

Diagnosis

■ PCR, serology or Tzanck smear

Treatment

ORAL ACYCLOVIR INDICATIONS:
■ More than 13 years of age (previously healthy child)
■ Chronic cutaneous/pulmonary disorder
■ Receiving oral or inhaled steroids or salicylates

INTRAVENOUS ACYCLOVIR INDICATIONS:
■ Immunocompromised
■ Severe disease
(encephalitis/pneumonia/hepatitis)

Immunoprophylaxis

Must be given within 96 hours of exposure

CANDIDATES FOR IMMUNOPROPHYLAXIS
■ Immunocompromised without history of varicella
■ Pregnant women
■ Newborns whose mother had an onset of chickenpox within 5 days before or 2 days after delivery
■ All preterm infants less than 28 weeks or less than 1000 gm
■ Preterm infants more than 28 weeks whose mother has no history of chickenpox or is seronegative

Vaccination

■ **Contraindicated** in immunocompromised (including HIV)

Complications

■ Pneumonia
■ Encephalitis/ataxia
■ Secondary bacterial skin infections

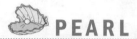

PEARL

In the immunocompromised, the lesions are often deep-seated, larger and umbilicated. Treat with VZIG.

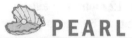

PEARL

AAP **does not recommend** treating uncomplicated varicella with acyclovir in healthy children.

Lyme Disease

Etiology

- *Borrelia burgdorferi* (deer tick—vector)

Manifestations

EARLY LOCALIZED PHASE (7 TO 14 DAYS AFTER BITE)
- Erythema chronicum migrans **("bulls eye rash")**

EARLY DISSEMINATED PHASE (DAYS TO WEEKS AFTER BITE)
- Seventh nerve palsy
- Aseptic meningitis
- Carditis **(heart block)**

LATE PHASE (WEEKS TO MONTHS AFTER BITE)
- **Arthritis** of large joints (knees)
- Polyneuritis

Diagnosis

- Serology

Treatment

EARLY PHASES AND ARTHRITIS
- Amoxicillin (less than 8 years old)
- Doxycycline (more than 8 years old)

MENINGITIS AND CARDITIS
- Intravenous ceftriaxone
- Intravenous penicillin G

Prognosis

- Excellent

CSF Characterization in Meningitis Infections

TYPE	CELL TYPE	PROTEIN	GLUCOSE
Bacterial	Neutrophils (300–2000 cells/mm³)	Elevated	Low
Viral	Lymphocytes (50–1000 cells/mm³)	Normal/increased	Usually normal
TB	Lymphocytes (10–500 cells/mm³)	Elevated	Low
Fungal	Lymphocytes (5–500 cells/mm³)	Elevated	Low

Infant Botulism

Organism

■ *C. botulinum*

Pathophysiology

■ Neurotoxin binds to presynaptic nerve terminals
■ Irreversible binding

Etiology

■ Ingestion of spores from **honey,** dust or soil

Manifestations

■ **Constipation**
■ Symmetric progressive weakness over days to weeks
■ Decreased suck, cry and flat facial expression
■ Ocular palsies
■ Autonomic abnormalities

Diagnosis

■ Stool for botulinum toxin

Treatment

■ **Human-derived botulinum anti-toxin**
■ Supportive

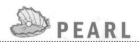 **PEARL**

Infants should not be fed honey until more than 12 months of age.

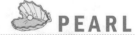 **PEARL**

Werdnig-Hoffman (spinal muscular atrophy) will also present with poor suck, decreased tone but will have *tongue fasciculations*.

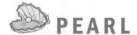 **PEARL**

Aminoglycosides are contraindicated because they may potentiate neuromuscular blockade.

Upper Airway Obstruction

TRACHEITIS

Etiology

- *S. aureus* (most common)
- *M. catarrhalis*
- Anaerobes

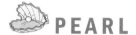

Manifestations

- **Toxic appearance**
- High fever
- Stridor
- **"Brassy" cough**
- Copious secretions

Treatment

- IV antibiotics (penicillinase-resistant penicillin)
- Humidification
- Oxygen

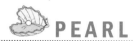

RETROPHARYNGEAL ABSCESS

Etiology

- Usually complication of bacterial pharyngitis

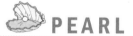

Manifestations

- High fever
- Difficulty swallowing
- Noisy breathing/hyperextended neck
- Drooling

Diagnosis

- Lateral neck radiograph: **widened retropharyngeal space**

Treatment

- IV antibiotic (must cover for *S. aureus*)
- Surgery

Upper Airway Obstruction

EPIGLOTTITIS

Etiology
- *H. influenzae* type b (**unimmunized child**)

Manifestations
- **Toxic appearance**
- Rapid progressive respiratory demise
- High fever
- Drooling/dysphagia
- **Neck hyperextension**

Neck Radiograph
- **"Thumb sign"** indicates swollen epiglottis

Diagnosis
- All suspected cases taken directly to operating room
- Do not attempt to exam anyone with suspected epiglottitis

Treatment
- Establish airway (intubation/tracheostomy)
- Intravenous antibiotics

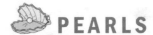

PEARLS

Classic position is **tripod**—sitting/leaning forward on arm with mouth open.

Peritonsillar abscess will present with trismus, drooling, **"hot potato voice,"** unilateral tonsillar swelling and a deviated uvula. Treatment is via needle aspiration and antibiotics.

REFERENCES

1. Shah B, Laude T: Atlas of Pediatric Clinical Diagnosis, 1st edition, Philadelphia, W.B. Saunders, 2000.

2. Behrman R, Kliegman R, Jenson H: Nelson Textbook of Pediatrics, 17th edition, Philadelphia, W.B. Saunders, 2003.

3. McMillan J, DeAngelis C, Feigin R, Warshaw J: Oski's Pediatrics—Principles and Practice, 3rd edition, Philadelphia, Lippincott, Williams & Wilkins, 1999.

4. Rudolph C, Rudolph A, Hostetter M, Lister G, Siegel N: Rudolph's Pediatrics, 21st edition, New York, McGraw-Hill, 2002.

5. AAP Red Book 2000, 25th edition, 2000.

MEDICATIONS

Medication Side Effects

AMINOGLYCOSIDES
- Nephrotoxicity
- Ototoxicity

AMIODARONE
- Pulmonary fibrosis
- Arrhythmias

AMPHOTERICIN
- Nephrotoxicity

ASPARAGINASE
- Pancreatitis

BLEOMYCIN
- Pulmonary fibrosis

CARBAMAZEPINE
- SIADH
- Ataxia/nystagmus (with use of erythromycin or verapamil)

CISPLATIN
- Nephrotoxicity

Medication Side Effects *continued*

CHLORAMPHENICOL
- "Gray baby" syndrome/aplastic anemia

CORTICOSTEROIDS
- Psychiatric symptoms
- Gastritis
- Myopathy (chronic)
- Osteoporosis/avascular necrosis
- Immunosupression
- Hyperglycemia
- Striae
- Hypertension
- Cataracts

CYCLOPHOSPHAMIDE
- Hemorrhagic cystitis

DOXORUBICIN
- Cardiac toxicity

FLUOROQUINOLONES
- Cartilage damage

FLUCONAZOLE
- GI symptoms/elevated liver enzymes

FUROSEMIDE
- Ototoxicity

HYDRALAZINE
- Drug-induced SLE

Medication Side Effects *continued*

INDOMETHACIN
- Closure of patent ductus arteriosus

KETOCONAZOLE
- Gynecomastia

METHOTREXATE
- Stomatitis/enteritis

MINOCYCLINE
- Pseudotumor cerebri

MONOAMINE OXIDASE INHIBITORS
- Hypertensive crises with tyramine (cheeses)

NSAIDS
- Peptic ulcer
- Gastritis

PENICILLIN
- Hypersensitivity reactions

PHENYTOIN
- Nystagmus
- Hirsutism
- Gingival hyperplasia

PROCAINAMIDE
- Drug-induced SLE

Medication Side Effects *continued*

SULFONAMIDES
- Photosensitivity
- Stevens-Johnson syndrome
- Hemolysis with glucose-6 phosphate deficiency

TETRACYCLINE
- Tooth discoloration
- Photosensitivity
- Pseudotumor cerebri (with isotretinoin)

THIAZIDES
- Hyponatremia

VANCOMYCIN
- "Red man syndrome" (histamine release—**no allergy**)

VINCRISTINE
- SIADH

Congenital Anomalies Associated with Medications

VALPROATE

- Narrow bifrontal diameter/high forehead
- Low nasal bridge/midfacial hypoplasia
- Cardiovascular anomalies (coarctation of aorta)
- Cleft lip
- Meningomyelocele

HYDANTOIN

- **Nail/digit hypoplasia**
- Developmental delay/mental deficits

RETINOIC ACID

- Facial asymmetry
- Hydrocephalus
- Microcephaly
- Microtia or anotia
- Conotruncal cardiac abnormalities

LITHIUM

- **Ebstein anomaly**

ACE INHIBITORS

- Fetal oligohydramnios
- Neonatal anuria
- Hypotension

WARFARIN

- Nasal hypoplasia
- Stippled epiphyses

Medications for Infections

INFECTION	MEDICATION
Oral cavity (dental abscess)	Penicillin
Osteomyelitis (> 5 years old)	Nafcillin Cephalothin Clindamycin (penicillin allergy)
Pneumococcal infections in sickle cell patient	Vancomycin
Skin infections	First-generation cephalosporins Cephalexin
Pseudomonas	Ceftazidime
Chlamdyia pneumonia	Erythromycin Clarithromycin Azithromycin
Mycoplasma pneumonia	Erythromycin Clarithromycin Azithromycin
Bites from humans, cats and dogs	Amoxicillin-clavulanate

REFERENCES

1. Taketomo C, Hodding J, Kraus D: Pediatric Dosage Handbook, 7th edition, Cleveland, Lexi-Comp Inc, 2000–2001.

2. Behrman R, Kliegman R, Jenson H: Nelson Textbook of Pediatrics, 17th edition, Philadelphia, W.B. Saunders, 2003.

3. McMillan J, DeAngelis C, Feigin R, Warshaw J: Oski's Pediatrics—Principles and Practice, 3rd edition, Philadelphia, Lippincott, Williams & Wilkins, 1999.

4. Rudolph C, Rudolph A, Hostetter M, Lister G, Siegel N: Rudolph's Pediatrics, 21st edition, New York, McGraw-Hill, 2002.

NEONATOLOGY

Children of Diabetic Mothers

Labs

- **Polycythemia** (hematocrit > 65%)
- Hyperinsulinemia
- **Hypoglycemia**
  - —Glucose < 35 mg/dl in term
  - —Glucose < 25 mg/dl in preterm
- Hypomagnesemia (magnesium < 1.5 mg/dl)
- Hypocalcemia (serum calcium < 7 mg/dl)

Maternal Complications

- Polyhydramnios
- Preeclampsia/preterm labor

Congenital Malformations

CARDIOVASCULAR
- Cardiomegaly
- VSD/ASD, transposition of arteries, coarctation of aorta
- Renal vein thrombosis—secondary to polycythemia

GASTROINTESTINAL
- Duodenal atresia
- **Hypoplastic left colon syndrome**
  -Stooling in 48 hours; usually no intervention needed

CENTRAL NERVOUS SYSTEM
- Jumpy/hyperexcitable
- Neural tube defect

MUSCULOSKELETAL
- **Large/plump at birth**
- Lumbosacral agenesis

Treatment

- Monitor blood glucose every hour for first 8 hours of life

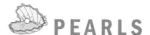

PEARLS

Hypocalcemia can be intractable unless hypomagnesemia is corrected.

Polycythemia is associated with lethargy, hypotonia, hypoglycemia and thrombocytopenia. Polycythemia is treated with phlebotomy with replacement saline or a partial exchange transfusion.

Bilious Vomiting in Newborn

Differential Diagnosis

- **Malrotation with/without volvulus** (most common)
- Duodenal web
- Intestinal atresia
- Annular pancreas
- Hirschsprung disease
- Meconium plug/ileus
- Necrotizing enterocolitis
- Duplication

Maternal History

- **Polyhydramnios**—intestinal atresia is highly suspected

Work-up

ABDOMINAL RADIOGRAPH STUDIES
- Upper GI study (**bird's beak** with volvulus)
- Malrotation has an **airless rectum**
- Duodenal atresia has a **double-bubble sign**
- Normally, air should be seen in the rectum of a healthy infant in the first 24 hours of life

Treatment

- Nasogastric tube
- Intravenous fluids
- Surgery

Neonatal Terminology

SMALL FOR GESTATIONAL AGE (SGA)   Weight $< 10^{th}$ percentile

APPROPRIATE FOR GESTATIONAL AGE (AGA)   Weight $> 10^{th}$ and $< 90^{th}$ percentile

LARGE FOR GESTATIONAL AGE (LGA)   Weight $> 90^{th}$ percentile

LOW BIRTH WEIGHT   Weight $> 1,500$ gm but $< 2,500$ gm

VERY LOW BIRTH WEIGHT   Weight $> 1,000$ gm but $< 1,500$ gm

EXTREMELY LOW BIRTH WEIGHT   Weight $< 1,000$ gm

Antepartum Terminology

LATE DECELERATIONS

A decrease in the fetal heart rate that begins after the peak of the uterine contraction; secondary to **decreased placental perfusion** during uterine contraction (associated with fetal hypoxia)

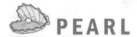 PEARL

A sign of **fetal distress.**

EARLY DECELERATIONS

A decrease in the fetal heart rate that begins with the onset of the uterine contraction; secondary to increased vagal tone from **increased fetal cranial pressure** due to the contraction

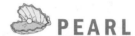 PEARL

Not a sign of fetal distress.

VARIABLE DECELERATIONS

Variable onset and duration fetal heart rate decelerations that differ in amplitude, duration and resolution; can occur between contractions (**associated with cord compression**)

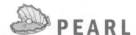 PEARL

Not a sign of fetal distress.

BEAT-TO-BEAT VARIABILITY

Instantaneous changes in the fetal heart rate

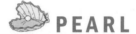 PEARL

Loss of beat-to-beat variability is associated with **fetal distress,** hypoxia, anemia or narcotics.

TACHYCARDIA (HEART RATE > 160 BEATS/MIN)

Associated with maternal fever, fetal hypoxia, maternal hyperthyroidism, beta-sympathomimetics, fetal anemia or fetal arrhythmias

BRADYCARDIA (HEART RATE < 120 BEATS/MIN)

Associated with fetal hypoxia, anesthetics, beta-blockers or heart block

Group B Streptococcal Infection

EARLY-ONSET

Timing
- Usually begins within 24 hours (0–6 days)

Manifestations
- **Pneumonia** (most common)
- Septicemia
- Meningitis

Labs
- Neutropenia
- Increased bands ($>$ **0.2 ratio of bands/neutrophils**)

Treatment
- Penicillin G and an aminoglycoside until GBS identified

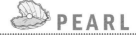

PEARL

Respiratory distress from group B streptococcal (GBS) pneumonia is indistinguishable from respiratory distress syndrome (RDS) due to surfactant deficiency. Use WBC (band/neutrophil ratio) to help differentiate between GBS from RDS; *cannot* use chest radiographs, ESR or ABGs.

LATE-ONSET

Timing
- 7 days to 3 months

Manifestations
- **Bacteremia without a focus** (most common)
- **Meningitis**
- **Osteomyelitis**

Labs
- Neutropenia
- ncreased bands ($>$ **0.2 ratio of bands/neutrophils**)

Treatment
- Penicillin G and an aminoglycoside until GBS identified

Congenital Syphilis

Manifestations

EARLY (APPEAR < 2 YEARS OLD)
- Hepatosplenomegaly
- Lymphadenopathy
- **"Snuffles"**
- **Thrombocytopenia**
- Osteochondritis
- Dermatologic
  - Copper-colored maculopapular lesion on hands and feet
  - Diffuse vesicobullous rash
  - Condyloma lata

LATE (APPEAR > 2 YEARS OLD)
- **Saddle nose**
- **Hutchinson teeth**/mulberry molars
- **Saber shins** (bowing of the tibia)

Diagnosis
- Serology/dark-field microscopy
- Long bone radiograph
- CSF VDRL

Treatment
- Penicillin

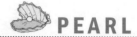

Must have high index of suspicion in mothers with history of STDs, multiple sex partners and drug abuse.

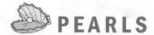

Asymptomatic infants at risk for syphilis include those treated less than 30 days before delivery and mother treated with erythromycin.

The **Jarisch-Herxheimer reaction** (fever, hypotension, tachycardia, chills and myalgias) can occur with treatment and is not an allergic reaction. Treatment should continue accordingly.

Congenital Toxoplasmosis

Etiology

- *Toxoplasma gondii* (transmitted via **cat stools**)

Manifestations

- **Asymptomatic at birth**
- Hepatosplenomegaly
- Lymphadenopathy
- Chorioretinitis
- **Intracranial calcifications**
- Hydrocephalus (**macrocephaly**)

Complications

- Blindness
- Mental retardation
- Learning disability
- Deafness

Diagnosis

- Serology

Treatment

- All infants treated with pyrimethamine.

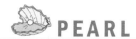

PEARL

Susceptible pregnant women should not handle cat litter.

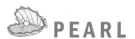

PEARL

Congenital CMV also has calcifications but is associated with microcephaly.

Neonatal Jaundice Pearls

- Jaundice occurring in the first 24 hours of life must be addressed as soon as possible. Etiologies include:

Elevated Direct Bilirubin	**Elevated Indirect Bilirubin**
TORCH infections	Erythroblastosis fetalis
Sepsis	

- Physiologic jaundice typically presents on the second or third day of life. Other etiologies of indirect jaundice that can present at this time include breast-feeding jaundice, delayed cord clamping, hematoma (from birth trauma).

- Physiologic jaundice is due to increased breakdown of fetal red blood cells and decreased conjugation in the liver.

- **Breast-feeding jaundice** is due to dehydration or reduced caloric intake and occurs in the first week of life. Need to increase feedings. Avoid supplementing with dextrose or water; may increase bilirubin levels.

- Must consider infections (UTI/sepsis) if jaundice appears after the third day of life (in first week of life)

- Etiologies if jaundice appears after the first week:

Elevated Direct Bilirubin	**Elevated Indirect Bilirubin**
Biliary atresia	Hypothyroidism
Sepsis	Breast milk jaundice
Hepatitis	Spherocytosis
Sepsis	Crigler-Najjar

- **Breast milk jaundice** typically presents in the second week of life and is due to an exaggerated enterohepatic circulation due to beta-glucuronidase in the milk. Self-resolving over time.

- Treatment of jaundice in a 2 to 3-day-old child is **phototherapy** for an indirect bilirubin $\geq$ 15 but < 25. If indirect bilirubin is $\geq$ 25, the treatment is an **exchange transfusion**.

Neonatal Resuscitation

- Infant placed on radiant warmer
- Dried quickly with towel
- Mouth is suctioned *first,* then nose
- If apnea or heart rate $<$ 100 begin positive-pressure ventilation with 100% oxygen and ventilate with bag mask for 15 to 30 seconds
- If heart rate does not increase after 15 to 30 seconds with bag-mask ventilation and the heart rate is $<$ 60 beats/min or if heart rate is $<$ 80 beats/minute and not rising, continue bag mask ventilation and begin chest compressions

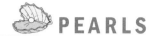 **PEARLS**

Consider naloxone in infant with depressed respiratory effort if there is a maternal history of narcotic analgesic use.

Newborns of mothers treated with magnesium sulfate can present with respiratory/motor depression and ileus.

Ritodrine/terbutaline can cause neonatal hypoglycemia, which is treated with 2 ml/kg of $D_{10}W$ followed by a continuous infusion at 6 to 8 mg/kg/min.

The use of naloxone in the delivery room is contraindicated in infants born to narcotic-addicted mothers because it may cause seizures.

The opening pressures to inflate airless lungs for the *first time* is higher than normally needed and is between 10 to 50 cm H_2O.

Neonatal Chest Radiographs

MECONIUM ASPIRATION

- **Coarse, diffuse, bilateral infiltrates** with irregular densities of consolidation with hyperinflated lungs

HYALINE MEMBRANE DISEASE

- **Diffuse reticulogranular pattern** in both lung fields with superimposed air bronchograms

TRANSIENT TACHYPNEA OF THE NEWBORN

- Clear lungs with prominent pulmonary vascular markings; **fluid lines in fissures and hyperaeration**

PATENT DUCTUS ARTERIOSUS

- Cardiomegaly

BIRTH ASPHYXIA

- Cardiomegaly

CHILD OF DIABETIC MOTHERS

- Cardiomegaly

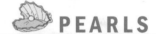 **PEARLS**

The Apgar scores (1 and 5 minutes) do not predict neonatal mortality or cerebral palsy. Actually, most patients who develop cerebral palsy have normal Apgar scores.

A score of ≤ 3 at 15 minutes has been associated with mortality and neurologic injuries.

If the Apgar score is ≤ 3 at 1 minute, resuscitation should be initiated.

If the 5-minute Apgar is < 7, it should be repeated every 5 minutes until it is > 7 or the child is 20 minutes old.

Apgar Scores

SIGNS	0 POINTS	1 POINT	2 POINTS
Heart rate	None	< 100/min	> 100/min
Respiration	None	Weak cry	Vigorous cry
Muscle tone	None	Some extremity flexion	Arms, legs well flexed
Reflex irritability	None	Grimace	Cough or sneeze
Color of body	Blue	Pink body/blue extremities	Pink all over

Herpes Simplex Infections

Etiology

- Usually with **primary maternal infection** (50% risk)
- 1 to 3% risk with recurrent exacerbations

Manifestations

DISSEMINATED (25%)
- Usually first few days of life
- Liver and adrenals are primary organs
- Sepsis-like picture

CENTRAL NERVOUS SYSTEM (35%)
- Presents in second to third weeks of life
- Seizures, lethargy
- CSF with elevated protein and mild pleocytosis

SKIN, EYES AND MOUTH (40%)
- Usually diagnosed in first 2 weeks of life
- Vesicles
- Often at trauma sites (i.e., scalp monitor)

Prognosis

DISSEMINATED
- Mortality: 60% (most common cause is **pneumonitis**)

CENTRAL NERVOUS SYSTEM
- Mortality: 15%
- 65% of survivors have neurologic impairment

Diagnosis

- CSF PCR
- Culture (skin, nasopharynx, eyes, stool, urine, blood)

Treatment

- IV acyclovir

Diaphragmatic Hernia

Pathophysiology

- Defect of posterolateral lumbosacral triangle (90%)

Manifestations

NEONATAL
- Severe respiratory distress
- **Pulmonary hypertension**

OLDER CHILDREN
- May be an **incidental finding** on chest radiograph

Diagnosis

- Usually via prenatal ultrasound

Treatment

- Supportive
- Extracorporeal membrane oxygenation (before/after repair)
- Surgical repair

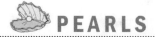

PEARLS

Look for loops of bowel in chest on chest radiograph.

Associated with **scaphoid abdomen** with decreased breath sounds or bowel sounds in the chest.

Retinopathy of Prematurity (ROP)

Risks

- **Low birth weight** (high risk for < 1500 gm)
- **Gestational age** (high risk for infants born < 33 weeks)
- **Hyperoxia**
- Multiple births

Exams

- Initial exam done at 4 to 6 weeks of age

Prognosis

AT RISK FOR:
- Myopia
- Strabismus
- Amblyopia
- Retinal detachment
- Blindness

Neonatal Cytomegalovirus

Manifestations

- **Asymptomatic** (>90%)
- Hepatosplenomegaly
- Purpura ("blueberry muffin" baby)
- Retinitis
- **Intracranial calcifications**
- **Microcephaly**

Complications

- Learning disabilities
- **Sensorineural deafness**
    - −60% of symptomatic infections
    - −15% of asymptomatic infections

Diagnosis

- PCR
- Serology (fourfold increase in titers)

Treatment

- Usually not treated

Necrotizing Enterocolitis

Etiology
PREDISPOSING FACTORS
- Prematurity
- Oral feeding/rapid feeding protocol
- Infectious agents? (occurs in epidemics)

Epidemiology
- Usually in the first 2 weeks of life

Manifestations
- **Abdominal distention**
- **Bloody diarrhea**
- Increased gastric residuals
- Sepsis-like picture/shock

Radiologic Findings
ABDOMINAL FILM
- **Pneumatosis intestinalis** (gas in the bowel wall)
- **Portal vein gas**
- Pneumoperitoneum
- Fixed dilated bowel (single/multiple loops in RLQ)

Treatment
- Cessation of feeds
- IV fluids
- Blood cultures
- IV antibiotics (i.e., ampicillin and aminoglycoside)
- Surgery consult

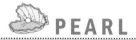

PEARL

Need a high index of suspicion, especially in symptoms starting after the initiation of feeds.

Fetal Alcohol Syndrome

Manifestations

FACIAL
- Microcephaly
- Short palpebral fissures
- Epicanthal folds
- Midfacial hypoplasia
- Short nose
- Long philtrum

CARDIAC
- Septal defects

CENTRAL NERVOUS SYSTEM
- Mental impairment
- Developmental delay

JOINTS
- Restriction of movement

Respiratory Distress Syndrome

Etiology
- Deficiency of surfactant in lungs

Manifestations
- Grunting
- Tachypnea
- Nasal flaring
- Chest retractions

Radiographic Findings

Reticulogranular pattern with air bronchograms
- "Ground glass" pattern

Treatment
- Oxygen
- Ventilation
- **Surfactant replacement therapy**

Prevention
- Maternal corticosteroids
    - −48 hours before preterm delivery (24–34 weeks)

Congential Torticollis

Etiology

- Intrauterine compression
- Trauma with birthing process
- Cervical vertebrae anomalies

Manifestations

- Head tilts to side of sternocleidomastoid muscle damage
- Chin will point to opposite side of involvement

Treatment

- Stretching
- Surgical release (if no improvement by 18 months old)

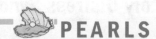

PEARLS

Radiographs of the cervical spine must be done prior to stretching treatment if no evidence of birth trauma or intrauterine compression is evident.

Klippel-Feil Syndrome (triad of short neck, low hairline and decreased neck mobility due to fusion of the cervical vertebrae) can present with torticollis; 40% of these patients have genitourinary tract abnormalities.

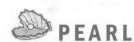

PEARL

An "olive mass" on the sternocleidomastoid muscle is seen secondary to birth trauma.

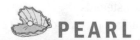

PEARL

CNS neoplasms are associated with acquired torticollis.

Erb and Klumpke Palsy

ERB PALSY

Etiology
- Traction injury to the upper brachial plexus
- Usually secondary to difficult labor and delivery

Injury Site
- C5, C6 and C7

Features
- **"Waiter's tip"**
- Shoulder adduction
- Internal rotation with wrist flexion
- Grasp reflex is *present* and biceps reflex is *absent*

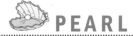 **PEARL**

C4 can be involved with **diaphragmatic paralysis** and respiratory distress. May show radiograph with one diaphragm higher than the other.

KLUMPKE PALSY

Etiology
- Traction injury to the lower brachial plexus
- Usually secondary to difficult labor and delivery

Injury Site
- C8 and T1

Features
- **Paralyzed hand**
- Good shoulder/elbow function
- Grasp reflex is *absent,* and biceps reflex is *present*

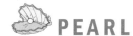 **PEARL**

Horner syndrome (miosis, partial ptosis, anhidrosis and enophthalmos) can occur secondary to cervical sympathetic nerve injury.

Apnea

ANEMIA OF PREMATURITY

- Anemia occurs at physiologic nadir (4–8 weeks)
- May be worsened by iron deficiency in rapidly growing preterm child
- Features: tachycardia

HYPOGLYCEMIA

- Usually occurs in preterm child immediately following birth
- Features: altered consciousness

INTRAVENTRICULAR HEMORRHAGE (IVH)

- Usually occurs in the first 7 days after birth
- Associated with infants requiring mechanical ventilation or with hemodynamic instability
- Features: hypotonia, decreased consciousness, posturing

SEPSIS

- Associated with indwelling catheters or endotracheal tubes

PATENT DUCTUS ARTERIOSUS

- Usually presents in the first 2 weeks of life
- Features: **widened pulse pressure,** bounding pulses, respiratory distress, tachycardia

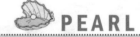 **PEARL**

Neonatal asphyxia initially causes gasping and irregular breathing, which should respond to stimulation/oxygen. However, if stimulation/oxygen is not given, apnea can develop that should be treated with positive pressure ventilation.

Antepartum Fetal Surveillance

NONSTRESS TEST

- Monitors the presence of fetal heart rate accelerations following fetal movement
- **"Reactive test"** is when two accelerations of the fetal heart rate occur in 20 minutes
- Reactive tests are associated with survival of the fetus for 1 week or more
- **"Nonreactive test"** is associated with poor outcomes in 20% of cases
- A nonreactive test requires additional evaluation, including a biophysical profile or a contraction stress test

CONTRACTION STRESS TEST

- Observes the fetal heart rate response to contractions (natural, oxytocin)
- If three contractions in 10 minutes are followed by late decelerations, it suggests fetal compromise
- **"Negative test"** is when no late decelerations were noted
- Contraindicated if history of premature rupture of membranes, placenta previa, prior uterine scar, multiple gestation, or incompetent cervix

BIOPHYSICAL PROFILE

- Observes fetus for movement, tone, reactivity, breathing and amniotic fluid
- Two points are given for each factor
- If 8 to 10 points, continue to monitor
- If 6 points, repeat biophysical profile in 24 hours
- If 0 to 4 points, consider delivery

Birth Trauma

CAPUT SUCCEDANEUM

- **Swelling crosses suture lines**
- Soft tissue swelling
- Resolves in days

CEPHALOHEMATOMA

- Subperiosteal
- Confined to **specific bones**
- 5% associated with linear, nondepressed skull fracture
- Associated with forceps delivery

SKULL FRACTURE

- Linear skull fractures do not need treatment; however, must be monitored for development of leptomeningeal cyst

CLAVICLE FRACTURE

- Present with **unilateral Moro reflex**

Risk Factors for SIDS

MATERNAL AND ANTENATAL RISK FACTORS

- Smoking
- Drug exposure
- Low socioeconomic status
- Fetal growth retardation

INFANT RISK FACTORS

- Prone sleep position
- Recent illness
- Smoke exposure
- Soft sleeping surface
- Age (2–4 months)

OTHER RISK FACTORS

- Cold season/climate
- Increased with blacks and Native Americans

REFERENCES

1. Shah B, Laude T: Atlas of Pediatric Clinical Diagnosis, 1st edition, Philadelphia, W.B. Saunders, 2000.

2. Behrman R, Kliegman R, Jenson H: Nelson Textbook of Pediatrics, 17th edition, Philadelphia, W.B. Saunders, 2003.

3. McMillan J, DeAngelis C, Feigin R, Warshaw J: Oski's Pediatrics—Principles and Practice, 3rd edition, Philadelphia, Lippincott, Williams & Wilkins, 1999.

4. Rudolph C, Rudolph A, Hostetter M, Lister G, Siegel N: Rudolph's Pediatrics, 21st edition, New York, McGraw-Hill, 2002.

5. AAP Red Book 2000, 25th edition, 2000.

NEPHROLOGY

Hematuria

IGA NEPHROPATHY—BERGER DISEASE

Etiology
- Uncertain; associated with prediagnostic viral infection

Manifestations
- **Gross/microscopic hematuria**
- Minimal proteinuria
- Elevated IgA
- **Normal complement**

Pathology
- IgA deposits in mesangium

Treatment
- Supportive

Prognosis
- Usually does not lead to significant kidney disease

POSTSTREPTOCOCCAL GLOMERULONEPHRITIS

Etiology
- Auto-antibodies

Manifestations
- Symptoms occur 1 to 2 weeks after streptococcal infection
- Tea-colored urine
- Hypertension
- **Low complement C3; normal C4**
- Edema
- **Microscopic/gross hematuria**
- Proteinuria
- Rare before 3 years old

Pathology
- "Humps" on epithelial side of basement membrane

Hematuria *continued*

Treatment
- Supportive

Prognosis
- Complete recovery (95%)

ALPORT NEPHRITIS

Etiology
- Autosomal dominant or X-linked dominant

Manifestations
- **Sensorineural deafness**
- **Gross/microscopic hematuria**
- Cataracts

Pathology
- Thinning, splitting, layering of basement membrane

Prognosis
- End-stage renal failure in second/third decade

IDIOPATHIC HYPERCALCIURIA

Etiology
- Idiopathic

Manifestations
- **Microscopic/gross hematuria**
- Nephrolithiasis

Diagnosis
- Check calcium-to-creatinine ratio of urine sample (> 0.2)
- 24-hour urine calcium excretion (> 4 mg/kg)

Treatment
- Thiazide diuretics
- Minimize oxalate-containing foods (chocolate, nuts, tea)

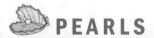 PEARLS

Avoid furosemide; it will *increase* calcium excretion.

Do not restrict calcium intake.

Minimum Change Disease

Etiology

- Unknown (frequently follows viral infection)

Epidemiology

- Males > females
- Usually between 2 to 8 years of age
- 80% of pediatric nephrotic syndromes

Manifestations

- **Edema**
- **Proteinuria**
- Hypoproteinemia
- **Elevated cholesterol**
- Decreased clotting factors
- Depleted intravascular volume

Pathology

- Retraction of foot process of epithelium

Treatment

- Sodium-restricted diet
- Initially **prednisone**
- Prednisone and cyclophosphamide (if refractory)
- Furosemdie/25% albumin with severe edema/ascites

Prognosis

- Usually full recovery

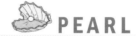

PEARL

Classic presentation is **periorbital edema**.

Metabolic Acidosis

Methanol poisoning
Uremia
DKA/diarrhea
Paraldehyde poisoning
Inborn errors of metabolism/ingestion of iron or isoniazid
Lactic acidosis
Ethanol poisoning/ethylene glycol poisoning
Salicylate toxicity/sepsis

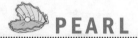 **PEARL**

Calculate the anion gap ($Na-(Cl-HCO_3)$) in metabolic acidosis. If **anion gap is less than 12** (hyperchloremic acidosis), the etiology is either diarrhea or renal tubular acidosis. If **anion gap is more than 12,** then etiology is one listed above in MUDPILES.

Renal Tubular Acidosis (RTA)

DISTAL RTA

- Failure to excrete hydrogen ions in the distal tubule
- Hypokalemia and hyperchloremia
- **High urine pH ($>$ 5.8) with severe systemic acidosis**
- Low serum bicarbonate

PROXIMAL RTA

- Reduced proximal tubular readsorption
- Severe bicarbonate wasting
- Associated with other urinary losses, including phosphate, glucose and amino acids
- Can occur alone or a with many other diseases, including Fanconi, cystinosis, medullary cystic disease, tyrosinemia or Lowe syndrome
- **Urine pH $<$ 5.5**

RTA IV

- End-organ resistance to aldosterone
- **Hyperkalemia, hyperchloremia metabolic acidosis**
- Positive urine anion gap
- Cannot generate ammonia
- Urine pH $<$ 5.5

Metabolic Alkalosis

URINE CHLORIDE < 10 MEQ/L

- Gastric losses (vomiting/nasogastric suction)
- Diarrhea
- Cystic fibrosis

URINE CHLORIDE > 10 MEQ/L

- Normal blood pressure
  - Bartter's syndrome
  - Acute diuretic use
- Hypertension
  - Cushing syndrome
  - Hyperaldosteronism

Hypernatremia

Definition

- Na > 150 mEq/L

Etiology

EXCESS OF SODIUM
- Formula mixing error
- Ingestion of sea water
- Excessive NAHCO$_3$ during resuscitation

WATER DEFICIT
- **Gastroenteritis/dehydration (diarrhea and poor intake)**
- Diabetes insipidus
- Inadequate breast feeding in a newborn

Treatment

- Slow rehydration over 48 to 72 hours for dehydration
- Lower sodium by 10 mEq/L in 24 hours
- Peritoneal dialysis if Na > 200 mEq/L

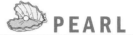

PEARL

Lithium is a cause of diabetes insipidus.

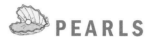

PEARLS

Rapid rehydration predisposes to cerebral edema and seizures.

Hyponatremia

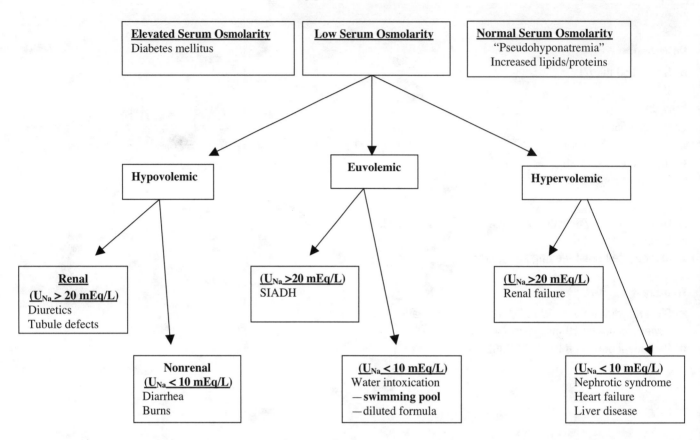

Elevated Serum Osmolarity	Low Serum Osmolarity	Normal Serum Osmolarity
Diabetes mellitus		"Pseudohyponatremia" Increased lipids/proteins

Hypovolemic → **Euvolemic** → **Hypervolemic**

Renal
($U_{Na} > 20$ **mEq/L**)
Diuretics
Tubule defects

Nonrenal
($U_{Na} < 10$ **mEq/L**)
Diarrhea
Burns

($U_{Na} > 20$ **mEq/L**)
SIADH

($U_{Na} < 10$ **mEq/L**)
Water intoxication
—**swimming pool**
—diluted formula

($U_{Na} > 20$ **mEq/L**)
Renal failure

($U_{Na} < 10$ **mEq/L**)
Nephrotic syndrome
Heart failure
Liver disease

Treatment

- Treat specific etiology accordingly
- Must correct slowly to avoid **central pontine myelinolysis**
- Adjust sodium about 10 to 12 mEq/L day
- Treat seizures/coma with 3% NaCl

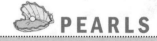

PEARLS

To diagnose hyponatremia etiology, use osmolarity and body volume status.

Rickets

DISEASE	DEFICIENCY	CALCIUM	PHOSPHATE	1,25-VITAMIN D	25-VITAMIN D	ALKALINE PHOSPHATASE
Vitamin D deficiency	Inadequate vitamin D or exposure to sunlight	Low-normal to low	Low	Low to normal	**Very low**	Elevated
Vitamin D dependent rickets— Type I	No 1 alphahydroxylase in kidney	Low	Low	**Extremely low**	Normal	Elevated
Vitamin D dependent rickets— Type II	End organ resistance to vitamin D	Low	Low or normal	**Extremely elevated**	Elevated	Elevated
Familial hypo-phosphatemia	Defect in conversion of 25 vitamin D to 1,25 vitamin D	Normal	Low	Low to low normal	Normal	Elevated

REFERENCES

1. Shah B, Laude T: Atlas of Pediatric Clinical Diagnosis, 1st edition, Philadelphia, W.B. Saunders, 2000.

2. Behrman R, Kliegman R, Jenson H: Nelson Textbook of Pediatrics, 17th edition, Philadelphia, W.B. Saunders, 2003.

3. McMillan J, DeAngelis C, Feigin R, Warshaw J: Oski's Pediatrics—Principles and Practice, 3rd edition, Philadelphia, Lippincott, Williams & Wilkins, 1999.

4. Rudolph C, Rudolph A, Hostetter M, Lister G, Siegel N: Rudolph's Pediatrics, 21st edition, New York, McGraw-Hill, 2002.

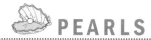 **PEARLS**

A board favorite radiograph of rickets will be an arm x-ray demonstrating the **cupping and fraying** of the distal ends of the radius and ulna.

Craniotabes occurs in rickets and is due to thinning of the outer skull; a "ping-pong" sensation is felt with palpation.

Palpable enlargement occurs at the junction of the rib and costochondral margins (**rachitic rosary**).

NEUROLOGY

Tuberous Sclerosis

Inheritance
- Autosomal dominant

Classic Triad
- Mental retardation
- Seizures (**infantile spasms**)
- Adenoma sebaceum (develop at 5 years of age)

Manifestations
- **Adenoma sebaceum** (mistaken for acne!)
- Shagreen patches (typically in thoracolumbar area)
- Cortical tubers (**calcifications**)
- Ungual fibromas
- Renal angiomyolipomas
- Renal cysts
- Cardiac rhabdomyomas
- Retinal hamartomas
- Hypopigmented macules (**ash leaf macules**)

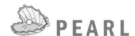

PEARL

Children with infantile spasm seizures must be considered for tuberous sclerosis.

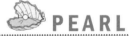

PEARL

Use Wood's lamp to identify ash leaf macules.

Rett Syndrome

Inheritance

- X-linked dominant

Gene Defect

- Gene encoding methyl-CpG binding protein 2

Manifestations

- Loss of milestones
- Seizures
- Spasticity
- Autistic behavior
- **"Hand wringing"**

Prognosis

- Death in adolescence

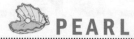

PEARL

Lethal in males; only occurs with females.

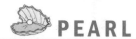

PEARL

Normal development until 1 year old, then motor and language milestones are lost.

Craniosynostosis

PRIMARY CRANIOSYNOSTOSIS

- Associated with a defect in **bone**
- *Unsymmetrically* shaped head
- Require surgical correction
- Associated with Apert and Crouzon syndromes

SECONDARY CRANIOSYNOSTOSIS

- Associated with a defect in the **central nervous system** (failure of brain to grow)
- *Symmetrically* shaped head
- Associated with mental retardation
- Does not require surgery, because brain growth usually does not occur

Febrile Seizures

SIMPLE CRITERIA

- **Tonic-clonic**
- $<$15 minutes
- Bilateral
- Self-limited

COMPLEX CRITERIA

- $>$15 minutes
- **Focal**
- Todd paralysis
- Repeated seizures in 24 hours

Prevalence

- 3% of children

Age

- 6 months to 5 years old

EEG

- Can be abnormal; does not have prognostic value

Treatment

- Diazepam to decrease recurrence risks

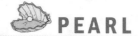

PEARL

Consider performing a lumbar puncture on children less than 12 months of age and children 12 to 18 months of age with fever/seizures because they may not exhibit classic meningitis signs.

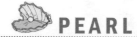

PEARL

Anticonvulsant prophylaxis is **not indicated** for simple febrile seizures.

Febrile Seizures *continued*

Recurrence of seizures

- 33%

Risk Factors

INCREASED WITH
- Family history
- Daycare attendance
- Neurologic anomaly

Recurrence Risk Factors

INCREASED WITH
- Age $<$ 12 months
- Seizure within the first 2 hours of fever
- History of febrile seizure in first-degree relative
- Complex seizures
- Seizures occurring at temperatures $<$ 40°C

Risk of Developing Epilepsy

- 1%

Epilepsy Risk Factors

INCREASED WITH
- Family history of epilepsy
- Febrile seizure at $<$ 9 months
- Prolonged or atypical febrile seizure
- Developmental delay
- Abnormal neurologic findings on exam

Neurofibromatosis (NF-1)

Inheritance

- Autosomal dominant

Diagnostic Criteria

TWO OR MORE OF THE FOLLOWING ARE NEEDED:

- Six or more *café au lait* macules
  - > 5 mm in prepubertal
  - > 15 mm in postpubertal
- ≥ 2 neurofibromas/one plexiform neurofibroma
- Axillary or **inguinal freckling**
- Optic glioma
- Two or more Lisch nodules
- Osseous lesions
- First-degree relative with NF-1

Complications

- Neurologic (seizures, learning disabilities)
- Psychological disturbances

Malignancy

INCREASED RISK OF A VARIETY OF TUMORS

- Neurofibrosarcoma
- Malignant schwannoma
- Wilms' tumor
- Pheochromocytoma
- Leukemia
- Rhabdomyosarcoma

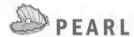 **PEARL**

At risk for hypertension secondary to **renal artery stenosis**.

Sturge-Weber Syndrome

Inheritance

■ Spontaneous

Manifestations

■ **Seizures** (90%)
■ **Port-wine stain** in first and second branches of trigeminal nerve (must cover at least one upper eyelid and forehead)
■ Venous leptomeningeal angiomatomas
■ Cognitive deterioration
■ Glaucoma

Diagnosis

■ MRI for leptomeningeal angiomatomas

Treatment

■ Partial hemispherectomy (improves outcome)
■ Monitor intraocular pressure

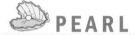 **PEARL**

Skull x-ray has **"railroad track"** appearance secondary to intracranial calcifications.

Guillain-Barré Syndrome

Pathophysiology
- Acute demyelinating condition of peripheral nerves
- Both motor and sensory affected

Etiology

2 TO 4 WEEKS AFTER
- Infection (CMV, EBV, HSV, *M. pneumoniae, C. jejuni*)
- Influenza or rabies immunization

Manifestations
- **Ascending paralysis over days**
- **Lower motor neuron condition**
- Reflexes are **absent**
- Paresthesias/weakness
- Respiratory compromise
- Autonomic abnormalities
    - —Hypertension/hypotension
    - —Cardiac arrhythmias

Labs

CEREBROSPINAL FLUID (CSF)
- **Elevated protein**
- Normal glucose
- Normal opening pressure
- **Normal WBC count**

Diagnostics
- Reduced nerve conduction velocity

Treatment
- **IVIG**
- Plasmapheresis
- Immunosuppressives
- Steroids

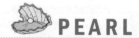

PEARL

Tick paralysis resembles Guillain-Barré, except ascending paralysis rapidly occurs over hours not days.

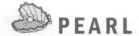

PEARL

Polyneuropathy with high CSF protein/no increased CSF WBC is diagnostic for Guillain-Barré.

Transverse Myelitis

Etiology
- Associated with preceding viral infections
- Can occur following rabies/smallpox vaccine

Manifestations
- **Abrupt onset** of lower extremity weakness
- Pain, temperature and light touch senses affected
- Upper motor lesion
- Fever
- Reflexes are **increased**
- **Loss of bladder control**

Diagnosis
- MRI of spinal cord

Treatment
- Supportive
- Usually resolves over weeks to months

Prognosis
- 10 to 15% have severe permanent neurologic deficits

Myasthenia Gravis

Pathophysiology

- Autoimmune attack on postsynaptic receptors

Manifestations

- **Weakness later** in the day
- Ptosis
- **Normal** reflexes

Labs

- Antibodies to acetylcholine receptors

Diagnosis

- **EMG**
- Antibodies to acetylcholine receptor

Treatment

- Neostigmine

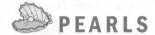 **PEARLS**

Infants born to mothers with myasthenia gravis (neonatal myasthenia gravis) present with respiratory distress, poor tone and suck. Symptoms resolve over days to weeks.

Congenital myasthenia gravis is a lifelong disease that does not have antibodies to acetylcholine receptors and is associated with significant ocular manifestations. Treatment is with cholinesterase-inhibiting drugs.

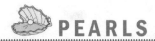 **PEARLS**

Cannot tolerate neuromuscular blockade drugs such as succinylcholine/pancuronium. If used, results in paralysis that last days to weeks.

Thymomas and Eaton-Lambert syndrome (associated with lung carcinoma) are not commonly seen in children as causes of myasthenia gravis.

Seizures

ROLANDIC SEIZURES

- Age of onset: 2 to 13 years of age
- 10% of epilepsy in school-age children
- Seizures are partial and involve the face, oral and buccal muscles
- Occur during the **sleep-awake transition**
- Prognosis: excellent
- Treatment: Anticonvulsants initially but usually can be discontinued

ABSENCE SEIZURES

- Occurs between 3 to 8 years of age
- More common in girls
- Seizures: **blank facies,** no motor activity; flickering of eyelids
- Seizure lasts 5 to 15 seconds and cause a brief decrease in consciousness
- EEG: **3-second spike and generalized wave**
- Hyperventilation induces seizure
- Treatment: ethosuximide

INFANTILE SPASMS

- Seizure: repetitive flexor/extensor spasms of neck, trunk and extremities
- Mental retardation
- EEG: **Hypsarrhythmia**
- Two types:
  - Cryptogenic—no cause identifiable (better prognosis)
  - Symptomatic—related to prenatal/perinatal factors
- Treatment: ACTH or valproic acid
- Prognosis: Poor; only 10 to 20% of infants achieve near normal development

JUVENILE MYOCLONIC EPILEPSY

- Seizure: initially is myoclonic jerks on awakening, **brushing teeth or combing hair**
- Over time develop into tonic-clonic generalized seizures
- Begins between 12 to 16 years of age
- 5 to 10% of epilepsy
- Treatment: valproic acid

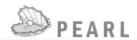 PEARL

May describe toothbrush or comb being dropped.

REFERENCES:

1. Shah B, Laude T: Atlas of Pediatric Clinical Diagnosis, 1st edition, Philadelphia, W.B. Saunders, 2000.

2. Behrman R, Kliegman R, Jenson H: Nelson Textbook of Pediatrics, 17th edition, Philadelphia, W.B. Saunders, 2003.

3. McMillan J, DeAngelis C, Feigin R, Warshaw J: Oski's Pediatrics—Principles and Practice, 3rd edition, Philadelphia, Lippincott, Williams & Wilkins, 1999.

4. Rudolph C, Rudolph A, Hostetter M, Lister G, Siegel N: Rudolph's Pediatrics, 21st edition, New York, McGraw-Hill, 2002.

NUTRITION

Effects of Excessive Vitamins and Nutrients

Vitamin A (Retinol)
- **Pseudotumor cerebri,** hepatosplenomegaly, bone pain
- Drying/cracking of skin, alopecia

Vitamin B$_6$ (pyridoxine)
- Sensory neuropathy

Vitamin C (ascorbic acid)
- Nausea, diarrhea, **nephrocalcinosis** (hyperoxaluria)
- Abdominal cramps

Vitamin D
- Anorexia, poor growth, **hypercalcemia,** polyuria and polydipsia

Vitamin E (tocopherol)
- No known toxic effects

Niacin (vitamin B$_3$)
- Skin flushing, itching

Effects of Deficiency of Vitamins

VITAMINS

Vitamin A (Retinol)
- Dermatitis, photophobia and **night blindness**

Vitamin B$_2$ (riboflavin)
- Photophobia, blurred vision, **glossitis**, cheilosis

Vitamin B$_6$ (pryridoxine)
- **Seizures**, dermatitis

Vitamin B$_{12}$ (cobalamin)
- Macrocytic anemia, neurologic deterioration

Vitamin C (ascorbic acid)
- Poor wound healing, **scurvy**, impaired collagen synthesis

Vitamin D
- Osteopenia and/or rickets

Vitamin E (tocopherol)
- Neurologic deficits of gait, spinocerebellar degeneration
- Decreased deep tendon reflexes and ocular palsy

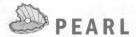 **PEARL**

Preterm formulas with high polyunsaturated fatty acids must have extra vitamin E added or **hemolytic anemia** can occur.

Effects of Deficiency of Nutrients

MINERALS

Thiamine (vitamin B$_1$)
- Beri beri (neuritis, congestive heart failure)

Zinc
ACRODERMATITIS ENTEROPATHICA
- **Perioral, perineal and acral rash**
- Sparse hair
- Chronic diarrhea/FTT
- Low zinc level
- Improves with age but may require zinc supplementation

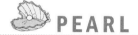 **PEARL**

Often presents when infant is weaned from breast milk to formula because human milk has a protein that facilitates zinc absorption.

Niacin (vitamin B$_3$)
- **Pellagra** (diarrhea, dermatitis and dementia)

Folic acid
- Macrocytic anemia, impaired growth

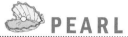 **PEARL**

Linolenic acid is an essential fatty acid. Children most at risk for deficiency include premature infants, children with fat malabsorption and those receiving long-term parental nutrition.

Selenium
- Cardiomyopathy

Linolenic acid
- Scaly dermatitis, hair loss, diarrhea and poor wound healing

Nutritional Value of Breast Milk Versus Cow's Milk

	BREAST MILK	COW'S MILK
Calories:	20 kcal/oz	20 kcal/oz
Total Protein:	Total: 1–1.5%	Total: 3.3%
Proteins:	70% Whey 30% Casein	20% Whey 80% Casein
Fat:	3.5%	3.5%
Carbohydrate:	Lactose	Lactose

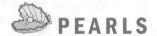

PEARLS

Cow's milk has a **greater** content of calcium, sodium, potassium and phosphorous than breast milk but **less** copper and iron.

Must supplement with vitamin D in strictly breast-fed infants to prevent rickets.

Kwashiorkor is a syndrome that occurs secondary to *protein deficiency* and presents with edema, hair loss, loss of muscle tone, dermatitis (pellagra-like rash) and increased infections.

Marasmus is due to *severe malnutrition* and presents with emaciation, loose skin, hypothermia, hypotonia and decreased activity.

Nutritional Value of Preterm Formula

Dilution
- 24 kcal/oz

Protein
- Whey:casein ratio of 60:40

Fat
- Medium-chain triglycerides

Carbohydrate
- Corn syrup solids

Calcium/Phosphorus Ratio
- 2:1

Trace Minerals
- Zinc
- Copper
- Selenium
- Chromium
- Manganese

REFERENCES

1. Behrman R, Kliegman R, Jenson H: Nelson Textbook of Pediatrics, 17th edition, Philadelphia, W.B. Saunders, 2003.

2. McMillan J, DeAngelis C, Feigin R, Warshaw J: Oski's Pediatrics—Principles and Practice, 3rd edition, Philadelphia, Lippincott, Williams & Wilkins, 1999.

3. Rudolph C, Rudolph A, Hostetter M, Lister G, Siegel N: Rudolph's Pediatrics, 21st edition, New York, McGraw-Hill, 2002.

4. Gunn V, Nechyba C: The Harriet Lane Handbook, 16th edition, Philadelphia, Mosby, 2002.

ONCOLOGY

Wilms' Tumor

Epidemiology
- Average age of diagnosis: 3 years old

Manifestations
- **Asymptomatic abdominal mass** (most common)
- Fever
- Hematuria
- Hypertension

Syndrome Associations

DENYS-DRASH
- Wilms' tumor
- Nephropathy
- Genitourinary abnormalities

WAGR
- Wilms' tumor
- Aniridia
- Genitourinary abnormalities
- Mental retardation

BECKWITH-WIEDEMANN
- Wilms' tumor
- Macroglossia
- Hemihypertrophy
- Visceromegaly

Initial Radiologic Study
- Ultrasound

Survival
- > 85% for stages I and II

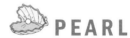 **PEARL**

CT scan findings of an *intrarenal tumor* usually rule out neuroblastoma.

Acute Lymphatic Leukemia (ALL)

Epidemiology

- Most common pediatric neoplasm

Manifestations

- Anorexia
- Fever
- Pallor/bleeding
- Splenomegaly
- **Bone/joint pain**

Radiographic Findings

- Transverse metaphyseal radiolucent bands
- Osteolytic lesions
- "Growth arrest lines"

Labs

- Pancytopenia

Diagnosis

- Bone marrow with **lymphoblasts**

Sites of Relapse

- Bone marrow (most common)
- CNS
- Testes

Cure Rate

- 80% (standard risk)

Risk Factors for Poor Outcomes

- **Age > 10 years old and < 1 year old**
- **High initial WBC count (> 50 X 10^9 L)**
- African American
- **Male**
- Poor response to initial induction chemotherapy
- Philadelphia chromosomes; t(9:22)

Complications

- Tumor lysis syndrome
    - —Associated with large tumor burden
    - —Phosphates, urates and potassium are released
    - —**Hyperphosphatemia causes hypocalcemia**
    - —Renal function can be compromised
    - —Treat with adequate hydration
    - —Uricase or allopurinol also used

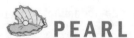

PEARL

Anemia and thrombocytopenia are present in 90% of cases.

Acute Lymphatic Leukemia (ALL) *continued*

Syndromes with Increased Risk of ALL

Down syndrome
Bloom syndrome
Severe combined immunodeficiency
Ataxia-telangiectasia
Neurofibromatosis
Wiskott-Aldrich

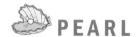

PEARL

Acute myeloid leukemia has **Auer rods** on blood smear.

Retinoblastoma

Age of Presentation
■ 13 to 18 months

Inheritance
■ Sporadically or autosomal dominant

Manifestations
■ **White pupillary reflex** (most common sign)
■ Strabismus

Prognosis
■ 90% for unilateral tumors

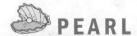

PEARL

All patients with **bilateral** disease have autosomal dominant disease along with 15% of those with unilateral disease.

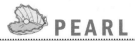

PEARL

Often diagnosed when a red reflex is not seen in a flash photograph of a child's face.

Pheochromocytoma

Pathogenesis
- Nonmalignant catecholamine-secreting tumor

Location
- Sympathetic ganglion chain
- Adrenal medulla (most common)

Presentation
- **Hypertension**
- Sweating/flushing
- Headaches (paroxysmal)
- Visual symptoms

Diagnosis
- Urine catecholamines (vanillylmandelic acid[VMA])
- Ultrasound
- **Radionucleotide scan with metaiodobenzylguanidine**

Treatment
TUMOR
- Removal of tumor is curative

HYPERTENSION
- Phenoxybenzamine (selective alpha-adrenergic blocker)
- Beta-blocker

Syndromes with Pheochromocytoma
- MEN IIA
- MEN IIB
- von Hippel-Lindau
- Neurofibromatosis

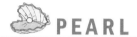

PEARL

Neuroblastoma also has elevated urine catecholamines and can also produce hypertension.

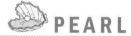

PEARL

Beta-blockers are *contraindicated* as lone medication because they would allow unopposed alpha effect and increase the blood pressure.

Neuroblastoma

Pathogenesis

■ Neural crest malignancy
■ Occurs along the sympathetic nervous system

Median Age of Diagnosis

■ 20 months

Manifestations

■ Neck mass
■ Flank or abdominal mass
■ Vasoactive intestinal peptide syndrome (watery diarrhea)
■ Periorbital ecchymoses; **"raccoon eyes"**
■ Opsoclonus-myoclonus; **"dancing eyes/dancing feet"**
■ "Blueberry muffin" nodules
■ Horner's syndrome
    —Miosis
    —Ptosis
    —Anhidrosis
    —Heterochromia of iris on affected side

Diagnosis

■ Biopsy
■ CT or MRI
■ Urine tumor markers
    —Vanillylmandelic acid (VMA)
    —Homovanillic acid (HVA)

Prognosis

■ < 1 year old; 95%

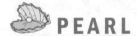

PEARL

Kidney is displaced (minimal distortion of calyceal system) with neuroblastoma, whereas Wilms' tumor is intrarenal and *distorts calyceal system*.

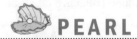

PEARL

Amplification of **n-*myc*** oncogene, **age greater than 2 years,** and bone metastases are associated with a poor prognosis.

Bone Tumors

OSTEOID OSTEOMA

- Benign
- Classic presentation is sharp, **boring pain that is worse at night** and relieved with aspirin or **nonsteroidals**
- 50% of time involves femur or tibia
- X-ray: radiolucent nidus with surrounding osteosclerosis
- Treatment: usually resolves; surgically removed if symptomatic

OSTEOCHONDROMAS

- Benign (most common benign bone tumor in children)
- Presents as a **painless, hard, nontender mass** of metaphysis of long bones
- X-Ray: bony outgrowth from the cortex
- Treatment: surgically removed if symptomatic

EWING'S SARCOMA

- Malignant
- Occurs in adolescents; *rare in African Americans*
- Presents with pain, swelling, and limitation of motion
- Systemic symptoms of **fever, fatigue and weight loss**
- Occurs in both extremity and central axis (flat bones/pelvis)
- X-ray: *onion-skin appearance;* lytic and destructive lesion with multilamellar periosteal reaction
- Treatment: chemotherapy, surgery and radiation

OSTEOGENIC SARCOMA

- Malignant (most common malignant bone tumor in children)
- Associated with radiation, Li-Fraumeni syndrome and hereditary retinoblastoma
- Occurs during adolescent growth spurt
- Presents with pain (nighttime awakening) and swelling
- **Systemic symptoms rare**
- Occurs in extremities in epiphysis/metaphysis of femur, tibia and humerus
- X-ray: lytic and blastic lesion
- Treatment: chemotherapy and surgery

Lymphoma

HODGKIN'S LYMPHOMA

- Bimodal occurrence: 15 to 30 years of age and more than 50 years old
- Presents as **firm, painless cervical/supraclavicular node** (most common)
- Fever, weight loss and night sweats (worse prognosis)
- Diminished cellular immunity
- Biopsy: **Reed-Sternberg cell**
- Treatment: Chemotherapy and radiation

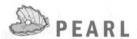

PEARL

Must consider Hodgkin's disease in previously healthy adolescent with opportunistic infection.

NON-HODGKIN'S LYMPHOMA (NHL)

- Neoplastic proliferation of immature lymphoid cells
- B-cell NHL commonly presents in abdomen
- T-cell NHL commonly presents in anterior mediastinum
- Most cases are very aggressive, show little differentiation and are highly malignant
- Risk factors include:
  - Congenital or acquired immunodeficiencies
  - EBV (Burkitt's lymphoma)
  - Wiskott-Aldrich syndrome
  - Severe combined immunodeficiency
  - Bloom syndrome
  - Ataxia telangiectasia

REFERENCES

1. Shah B, Laude T: Atlas of Pediatric Clinical Diagnosis, 1st edition, Philadelphia, W.B. Saunders, 2000.

2. Behrman R, Kliegman R, Jenson H: Nelson Textbook of Pediatrics, 17th edition, Philadelphia, W.B. Saunders, 2003.

3. McMillan J, DeAngelis C, Feigin R, Warshaw J: Oski's Pediatrics—Principles and Practice, 3rd edition, Philadelphia, Lippincott, Williams & Wilkins, 1999.

4. Rudolph C, Rudolph A, Hostetter M, Lister G, Siegel N: Rudolph's Pediatrics, 21st edition, New York, McGraw-Hill, 2002.

OPHTHALMOLOGY

Strabismus

Manifestations

- Esotropia: inward deviation of eyes
- Exotropia: outward deviation of eyes
- Hyperdeviation: upward deviation of eyes
- Hypodeviation: downward deviation of eyes

Diagnosis

CORNEAL LIGHT REFLEX
- Asymmetric corneal light reflex

COVER-UNCOVER TEST
- Affected eye will move to fixate on object after the unaffected eye is covered

ALTERNATE-COVER TEST
- Affected eye will move after cover is lifted to the other eye

Treatment

- Patching of the stronger eye
- Correction of refractive error with glasses
- Extraocular muscle surgery

Prognosis

- Untreated, child can develop **amblyopia**

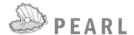 **PEARL**

Pseudostrabismus occurs in Asians and in children with Down syndrome.

Referral to Ophthalmologist

- Persistent abnormal head position
- Strabismus (infants > 6 months)
- Nystagmus
- Aversion to occlusion
- Abnormal red reflexes
- Persistent squinting
- Closing or covering one eye
- Abnormal vision acuity examination
  - 3.5 years old: 20/50 or worse in one or both eyes
  - > 5 years old: 20/40 or worse in one or both eyes

Ophthalmia Neonatorum

GONOCOCCAL CONJUNCTVITIS (*N. GONORRHOEAE*)

- Can be present at birth (premature rupture of membranes); typically 1 to 5 days of life
- Eye: bilateral, intense lid edema and **thick mucopurulent discharge**
- Associated with meningitis, septicemia and arthritis
- Gram stain: gram-negative intracellular **diplococci**
- Culture on Thayer-Martin chocolate agar
- Treatment: IV or IM ceftriaxone or cefotaxime
- Can lead to corneal ulcers, glaucoma or blindness
- Prophylaxis within 1 hour of birth: all infants receive either silver nitrate, erythromycin or tetracycline ointment
- Must suspect *C. trachomatis,* syphilis and/or HIV coinfection
- Mother and sexual partner must be evaluated for sexually transmitted diseases

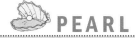

PEARL

Infants born to mothers with gonorrhea should receive a single day of parental antibiotics in addition to ocular prophylaxis.

CHLAMYDIA CONJUNCTIVITIS (*C. TRACHOMATIS*)

- Usually presents during first 1 to 2 weeks of life
- Most common infectious neonatal conjunctivitis
- Eye: bilateral, hyperemia of conjunctiva and mucopurulent discharge
- Associated with pneumonia/eosinophilia
- Giesma stain: **intracytoplasmic inclusion bodies**
- Diagnose with PCR, enzyme immunoassay or direct fluorescent antibody staining
- Treatment: erythromycin for 10 to 14 days
- Can lead to corneal scarring
- Must suspect *N. gonorrhoeae,* syphilis and/or HIV coinfection
- Mother and sexual partner must be evaluated for sexually transmitted diseases

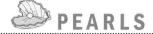

PEARLS

Prophylaxis medication for *N. gonorrhoeae* **does not** prevent chlamydial conjunctivitis.

Erythromycin increases risk of hypertrophic pyloric stenosis in infants less than 6 weeks of age.

Red Eye

INFECTIOUS

- Most common bacterial infection: *H. influenzae*
- Most common viral infection: adenovirus
- Viral infections frequently occur in fall/winter

Treatment
- Bacterial: topical antibiotic ointment
- Viral: cool compresses

ALLERGIC

- Seasonal exacerbations
- **Bilateral, itchy, watery discharge**
- Concurrent atopic disorder
- Treatment: ocular antihistamine

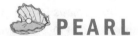

PEARL

Consult ophthalmology before treating any conjunctivitis with ocular steroids.

Infantile Glaucoma

Etiology

PRIMARY (50%)
- Defect of drainage in anterior chamber angle

SECONDARY (50%)
- Trauma
- Congenital rubella syndrome
- Sturge-Weber
- Neurofibromatosis
- Lowe syndrome
- Retinopathy of prematurity
- Marfan syndrome

Manifestations

- **Epiphora** (excessive tearing)
- **Photophobia**
- **Blepharospasm** (voluntary eyelid closure)
- Cloudy/white cornea
- Megalocornea (>10 mm in diameter)
- "Red eye"

Labs

- Elevated intraocular pressure (> 25 mmHg)

Complications

- Blindness
- Myopia

Treatment

- Surgical
- Carbonic anhydrase inhibitors
- Beta-blockers

White Pupillary Reflex

CATARACTS

- Genetic
- TORCH intrauterine infection
  - Toxoplasmosis
  - Varicella-zoster
  - Rubella
  - Cytomegalovirus
  - Herpes simplex
  - Rubeola
- Metabolic
  - Galactosemia
  - Diabetes mellitus
  - Alport syndrome
  - Lowe syndrome
- Chromosomal
  - Trisomy 21, 13, and 18

MALIGNANCY

- Retinoblastoma

INFECTIOUS

- Ocular larva migrans (*T. canis*)

OCULAR DISEASE

- Retinal detachment
- Retinal dysplasia

REFERENCES

1. McMillan J, DeAngelis C, Feigin R, Warshaw J: Oski's Pediatrics—Principles and Practice, 3rd edition, Philadelphia, Lippincott, Williams & Wilkins, 1999.

2. Nelson L: Harley's Pediatric Ophthalmology, 4th edition, Philadelphia, W.B Saunders, 1998.

3. AAP Red Book 2000, 25th edition, 2000.

4. Shah B, Laude T: Atlas of Pediatric Clinical Diagnosis, Philadelphia, W.B. Saunders, 2000.

5. Behrman R, Kliegman R, Jenson H: Textbook of Pediatrics, 17th edition, Philadelphia, W.B. Saunders, 2003.

ORTHOPEDICS

Adolescent Idiopathic Scoliosis

Screening
- Annually for all adolescents (especially females)

Examination
- Forward-bending examination (Adams' test)
- Can detect very small curvatures
- Asymmetry of posterior chest wall

Monitoring
LESS THAN 20-DEGREE CURVATURE
- Evaluate every 6 months in growing child

20 TO 30-DEGREE CURVATURE
- Evaluate every 3 months in *premenarchal* girls
- Evaluate every 6 months in more skeletally mature children

Treatment
NO TREATMENT
- If curves <**25 degrees**, regardless of age

BRACING
- Halts progression
- Immature adolescents with curve > 25 degrees but < 45 degrees

SURGERY
- Internal fixation rods and fusion
- Curve > **45 degrees**, regardless of age

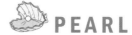 PEARL

Premenarchal girls are at **higher risk** of progression of curve than postmenarchal girls.

Subluxation of the Radial Head

Etiology

- Annular ligament slips into radiohumeral joint space
- **Painful**

Risk Factors

- Traction (pulling) of an extended/pronated arm

Manifestations

- Child will hold arm close to the body
- **Arm is pronated and slightly flexed**
- Child refuses to use hand of affected arm

Treatment

- Hold elbow at 90 degrees
- Manipulate forearm into supination

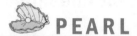 **PEARL**

Occurs with **swinging a child by arms** or lifting a child by an arm.

Fractures

Supracondylar
- Occurs with fall onto outstretched hand

Greenstick
- Incomplete fracture
- Occurs at the junction of the diaphysis and metaphysis.

Spiral
- Caused by twisting mechanism

Comminuted
- Contain multiple fragments

Toddler
- Spiral fracture
- Occur between 2 to 4 years of age
- Occur in distal third of tibia

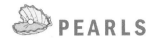

PEARLS

Look for **posterior fat pad** displacement on x-ray in supracondylar fractures.

Associated with vascular compromise.

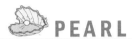

PEARL

Cortex/periosteum remain *intact* on one side in greenstick fractures.

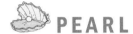

PEARL

Must rule out **child abuse** with spiral fractures.

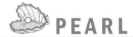

PEARL

Toddler's fractures are associated with **benign trauma,** such as a simple fall when running or playing.

Children with a Limp

LEGG-CALVÉ-PERTHES (AVASCULAR NECROSIS OF FEMORAL HEAD)

Age
- Usually 2 to 12 years old (mean: 7 years old)

Sex
- Males > females

Manifestations
- Typically **painless**
- Often follows a minor fall
- Mild abductor weakness
- Atrophy of thigh and gluteal muscles

Diagnosis
- Anteroposterior and frog-leg x-rays

Treatment
- Observation (all children < 6 years of age)
- Nonsurgical containment
- Surgery

SLIPPED CAPITAL FEMORAL EPIPHYSIS (SCFE)

Age
- Adolescence

Sex
- Males > females

Manifestations
- **Painful**
- **Obese** or **tall/thin adolescents** with recent growth spurt
- Externally rotated extremity

Diagnosis
- Anteroposterior and frog-leg X-rays

Treatment
- Surgical pinning

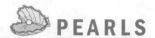 **PEARLS**

Patients with SCFE may complain only of **knee pain.**

When SCFE occurs before adolescence one must rule out an **endocrine disorder** (hypothyroidism, growth hormone deficiency).

Acute Hip Pain

TRANSIENT SYNOVITIS

- Commonly associated with a history of a recent URI
- Children **do not appear very ill**
- Fever may be present
- Leg will be held in flexion, abduction and externally rotated
- Usually normal to mildly elevated labs (ESR and WBC)
- Effusion/widened joint space may be noted on ultrasound
- Diagnosis is one of exclusion, if unsure, hip needs to be aspirated

SEPTIC ARTHRITIS

- Children **appear ill**
- Typically, hip involved in infants and knees in older children
- Swelling, warmth, and erythema on exam
- Limited range of motion of leg
- *S. aureus* most common organism
- Abnormal labs with **elevated WBC and ESR**
- Joint aspirate with elevated WBC 50,000 to 250,000 (95% PMNs)
- Surgical drainage and IV antibiotics are needed in all cases

Developmental Dysplasia of the Hip

Epidemiology
- Females more often than males
- Breech deliveries
- First-born children

Manifestations
- Barlow: posterosuperior hip dislocation with adduction
- Ortolani: **"clunk"** with abduction

Diagnosis
- Ultrasound
- Anteroposterior/frog-leg view x-ray in older children (> 6 months)

Treatment
NEONATE
- Pavlik harness

AGE 1 TO 6 MONTHS
- Pavlik harness
- Surgical closed reduction if harness fails

AGE 6 TO 18 MONTHS
- Surgical closed reduction

AGE >18 MONTHS
- Surgical open reduction

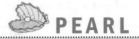

PEARL

Hip clicks are not necessarily pathologic and could be due to surface tension on hip joint, snapping gluteal tendons or from the patella.

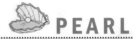

PEARL

X-ray will demonstrate a nonequal relationship between the femoral heads and acetabulum.

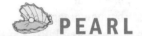

PEARL

Double-diapering is an ineffective form of treatment.

Orthopedic Pearls

METATARSUS ADDUCTUS

- In-toeing of the forefoot with normal hindfoot
- Secondary to intrauterine positioning (more common in first-born)
- Dorsiflexion and plantar flexion are *normal*
- Most resolve spontaneously
- Surgery rarely needed

TALIPES EQUINOVARUS (CLUB FOOT)

- Medial rotation of tibia, flexion at ankle with inversion of the foot and forefoot adduction
- Dorsiflexion and plantar flexion *are restricted*
- **Rigid foot**
- Treatment: serial casting and surgery

INTERNAL TIBIAL TORSION

- Most common cause of **in-toeing in children less than 2 years old**
- Associated with metatarsus adductus
- Resolves spontaneously
- Night splints are not recommended

INTERNAL FEMORAL TORSION

- Most common cause on **in-toeing in children more than 2 years old**
- Associated with generalized ligamentous laxity
- Affected children commonly sit in **"W" style**
- Resolves spontaneously
- Night splints are not recommended

GENU VARUM (BOWLEGS)

- Differential diagnosis:
  - Physiologic
  - Tibia vara (abnormal growth of tibial epiphysis)
  - Rickets

- **Treatment**
  - Physiologic—observation
  - Tibia vara—observation and/or surgery
  - Rickets—nutritional

Orthopedic Pearls

IDIOPATHIC KYPHOSIS (SCHEUERMANN'S DISEASE)

- Nonflexible kyphosis
- Develops in adolescence
- Individuals cannot actively correct the defect
- Treatment varies from exercises, bracing or surgery

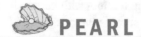

PEARL

Flexible kyphosis is differentiated from idiopathic kyphosis because the children can correct the defect in both standing and prone positions.

OSGOOD-SCHLATTER DISEASE

- Traction apophysitis
- Occurs at the insertion of the patellar tendon on the tibial tuberosity
- Associated with overuse of quadriceps muscle
- Typically presents in children from 10 to 15 years of age
- Manifests as pain, swelling of tibial tuberosity
- Pain with running, jumping and stair climbing
- Resolves when patient reaches skeletal maturity
- Treatment: stretching, Osgood-Schlatter pad and NSAIDS

PATELLOFEMORAL PAIN SYNDROME

- Most common cause of chronic anterior knee pain
- Worse with prolonged sitting, going up stairs or running
- Diagnosed via peripatellar tenderness or positive patella glide test
- Treatment includes anterior knee exercises, soft knee braces and NSAIDs

REFERENCES

1. McMillan J, DeAngelis C, Feigin R, Warshaw J: Oski's Pediatrics—Principles and Practice, 3rd edition, Philadelphia, Lippincott, Williams & Wilkins, 1999,

2. Behrman R, Kliegman R, Jenson H: Textbook of Pediatrics, 17th edition, Philadelphia, W.B. Saunders, 2003.

3. Beaty J, Kasser J: Fracture in Children, 5th edition, Philadelphia, Lippincott, Williams & Wilkins, 2001.

4. Herring J: Pediatric Orthopedaedics, 3rd edition, Philadelphia, W.B. Saunders, 2002.

PREVENTION

Cholesterol Screening

CRITERIA FOR TOTAL BLOOD CHOLESTEROL SCREENING

- Parent with cholesterol > 240 mg/dl
- Cigarette smoking
- High blood pressure
- Physical inactivity
- Severe obesity (>30% above ideal weight)

CRITERIA FOR FASTING LIPOPROTEIN SCREENING

- Patient cholesterol > 200 mg/dl
- Parent or grandparent with
  - Coronary atherosclerosis < 55 years old
  - Peripheral vascular disease < 55 years old
  - Cerebrovascular disease < 55 years old and cholesterol > 240 mg/dl

AAP Guidelines to Prevent Group B Streptococcal Infections

- All women should have anorectal and lower vaginal cultures done at 35 to 37 weeks' gestation.
- Indications **for intrapartum chemoprophylaxis** with IV penicillin G
  - History of previous infant with invasive group B streptococcus
  - Group B streptococcal bacteriuria during pregnancy
  - Preterm labor (< 37 weeks)
  - Fever ($> 38°C$)
  - Ruptured membranes greater than 18 hours
- Women positive for group B streptococcal infection may choose **intrapartum chemoprophylaxis.**

Hepatitis B Prophylaxis Following Percutaneous Blood Exposure

UNIMMUNIZED EXPOSED PERSON

- If source is HBsAg positive: give HBIG and start vaccine
- If source is HBsAg negative: start vaccine
- If source is unknown/not tested: start vaccine

IMMUNIZED EXPOSED PERSON (KNOWN RESPONDER)

- If source is HBsAg positive: no treatment
- If source is HBsAg negative: no treatment
- If source is unknown/not tested: no treatment

IMMUNIZED EXPOSED PERSON (KNOWN NONRESPONDER)

- If source is HBsAg positive: give two doses of HBIG or one dose of HBIG and restart vaccine
- If source is HBsAg negative: no treatment
- If source is unknown/not tested: give two doses of HBIG or one dose of HBIG and start vaccine if source considered high-risk (IV drug user)

IMMUNIZED EXPOSED PERSON (RESPONSE UNKNOWN)

- If source is HBsAg positive: test exposed for HBsAg antibody level
  - If low: one dose of HBIG and vaccine booster dose
  - If adequate: no treatment
- If source is HBsAg negative: no treatment
- If source is unknown/not tested: test exposed for HBsAg antibody level
  - If low: vaccine booster
  - If adequate: no treatment

Indications for Hepatitis A Vaccine

- Travel or working in a country with a high endemic rate of hepatitis A
- Children (> 2 years old) living in communities with high hepatitis A infection rates
- People with chronic liver disease (at risk for **fulminant hepatitis A**)
- Homosexual/bisexual men
- IV drug users
- Children with clotting-factor disorders
- Lab workers

Postexposure Immunoprophylaxis for Hepatitis A

IF EXPOSURE WAS IN THE LAST 14 DAYS

- Immunoglobulin for all patients
- If a future exposure is likely and patient is $\geq$ 2 years of age give hepatitis A vaccine

IF EXPOSURE WAS MORE THAN 14 DAYS AGO

- No prophylaxis (**immunoglobulin must be given within 2 weeks of exposure**)
- If a future exposure is likely and patient is $\geq$ 2 years of age, give hepatitis A vaccine

General Prevention Information

LEAD POISONING

■ Screen via capillary blood sample at 18 to 24 months.

CHILD PROOFING

■ Discussion on child proofing home should be done *before* child is mobile (i.e., at 6-month well child exam).

NEURAL TUBE DEFECTS

■ Pregnant women should take folate.

POOL DROWNING

■ The best method to prevent a drowning at a home pools is with a fence and locked gate.

DEVELOPMENTAL SCREENING

■ The primary goal of the developmental screening of young children by the general pediatrician is early identification of children who need further assessment.

THUMB SUCKING

■ Normal practice until the age of 4 years. Persistence after 4 years old can cause serious orthodontic problems. Efforts to discontinue thumb sucking should begin **after the age of 4.**

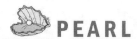

PEARL

Neural tube defects are also associated with diabetic mothers and fetuses exposed to valproic acid.

General Prevention Information

VIOLENCE

■ AAP recommends limit of 1 to 2 hours of television watching a day.

HYPERTENSION

■ Initiate routine screening of blood pressure at 3 years of age.

SUN EXPOSURE

■ 80% of a person's lifetime sun exposure occurs during the first two decades of life and if sunscreens are used they reduce the risk of skin cancer by 80%.

NEONATAL GONOCOCCAL CONJUNCTIVITIS

■ Topical silver nitrate, erythromycin and tetracycline ointment all prevent gonorrhea infections in newborns.

BEDWETTING AT SLEEPOVER

■ Give desmopressin via nasal spray at bedtime.

Transfusions

ALL BLOOD DONATED IN THE USA IS SCREENED FOR

- Antibodies to HIV
- HIV antigen
- Antibodies to human T-cell lymphotrophic virus
- Antibodies to hepatitis B core antigen
- Antibodies to hepatitis B surface antigen
- Antibodies to hepatitis C
- Syphilis

Car Seat Recommendations

INFANTS: < 20 LBS. AND < 1 YEAR OF AGE

- Rear-facing car seat in the middle of the back seat with infant at a 45-degree angle

WEIGHT: 20 TO 40 LB

- Forward-facing convertible car seat in middle of back seat

WEIGHT: 40 TO 60 LB

- Booster seat placed in back seat

WEIGHT: 60 TO 80 LB

- Standard seat belt but child should sit in back seat until the age of 12 years

Indications for Pneumovax

- Children older than 2 years of age with diseases that increase the risk of acquiring pneumococcal infection or significant disease if they become infected:
  - **Sickle cell disease**
  - Asplenia (functional or anatomic)
  - Nephrotic syndrome
  - Chronic renal failure
  - Immunosuppression secondary to transplantation
  - HIV
  - Cerebrospinal fluid leaks
- Children older than 2 years of age with cardiovascular, pulmonary or liver disease
- Children older than 2 years of age who live in settings with a high risk of invasive pneumococcal disease or its complications:
  - Alaskan natives
  - Native-American populations

Recommendations for Influenza Vaccine

- Children who are 6 months of age or older with one or more of the following:
  - Asthma
  - Cardiac disease
  - Immunodeficiency
  - HIV
  - Sickle cell anemia/hemoglobinopathies
  - Any disease the requires long-term aspirin therapy (juvenile rheumatoid arthritis or Kawasaki disease), which could increase the risk of Reye's syndrome following an influenza infection
- Children and adolescents at risks for complicated influenza, particularly those with the following disorders:
  - Diabetes mellitus
  - Renal disease
  - Metabolic disorders
  - Pregnancy (give vaccine in second or third trimester)

Normal Growth Parameters

HEAD CIRCUMFERENCE

- Average head circumference at birth: 34.8 cm
- Head circumference should increase by 0.5 cm/wk during the first 2 months of life and 0.25 cm/wk from 2 to 6 months of life

LENGTH

- Average length at birth: 50 cm
- Length should increase by 50% at 1 year, double by 4 years and triple by 13 years of life

WEIGHT

- Average weight at birth: 3.25 kg
- A newborn should gain 25 gm/day
- Weight should double by 5 months and triple by 1 year of life

REFERENCES

1. McMillan J, DeAngelis C, Feigin R, Warshaw J: Oski's Pediatrics—Principles and Practice, 3rd edition, Philadelphia, Lippincott, Williams & Wilkins, 1999,

2. Behrman R, Kliegman R, Jenson H: Textbook of Pediatrics, 17th edition, Philadelphia, W.B. Saunders, 2003.

3. Rudolph C, Rudolph A, Hostetter M, Lister G, Siegel N: Rudolph's Pediatrics, 21st edition, New York, McGraw-Hill, 2002.

PSYCHIATRY

Conversion Disorders

Pathophysiology
- A physical symptom that occurs following stress or conflict
- Loss of function or alteration **without organic etiology**
- Start suddenly/stop abruptly
- Not intentionally produced

Manifestations
- Blindness
- Deafness
- Seizures (**pseudoseizures**)
- Chest pain
- Abdominal pain
- Paralysis
- Weakness

Prognosis
- Rapid remission usually occurs.

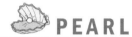 **PEARL**

Symptoms correlate with a friend/relative with similar symptoms of an actual illness.

Sleep Disorders

NIGHT TERRORS

- Child usually sits up in bed, appears frightened and anxious
- Pupils dilated
- Unresponsive to comfort efforts
- **Not remembered** upon awakening
- Begins between 4 and 12 years old
- Usually occur **1 to 2 hours** after falling asleep
- Occur in stages III–IV

NIGHTMARES

- Child is fearful, anxious and seeking comfort upon awakening
- **Remembered** upon awakening
- Occur in REM sleep
- Usually occur in the **second half** of the night
- Peak occurrence between 3 and 6 years old

NARCOLEPSY

- Often presents in adolescence
- Attacks of rapid eye movement sleep during wakefulness
- Excessive daytime sleepiness
- **Hypnagogic hallucinations** (frightening)
- **Cataplexy**—sudden inhibition of muscle group
- **Sleep paralysis**—occurs when falling asleep
- Treatment: stimulants

Attention Deficit Hyperactivity Disorder

Epidemiology

- 3-6% of school-age population
- Males more than females
- Occurs with oppositional defiant disorder/conduct disorder

Manifestations

- Trouble organizing
- Difficulty listening
- Fidgets
- Easily distracted
- Impulsive

Diagnosis

ESSENTIAL CRITERIA

- Impairment prior to the age of 7 and after 6 months
- Occurrence in **more than one setting**
- Impairment of social, academic or occupational functioning

Treatment

- Psychosocial interventions
- Pharmacologic
    Methylphenidate
    Dextroamphetamine

Prognosis

- 30 to 50% have symptoms as adults

Separation Anxiety Disorder

Definition
■ Anxiety when separated from home or parents

Manifestations
■ Unrealistic/persistent worries of harm coming to parents
■ **School avoidance**
■ Wanting to be near parents when sleeping
■ Avoidance of being alone
■ Somatic complaints

Treatment
■ **Early return to school**
■ Family therapy
■ Serotonin-uptake inhibitors

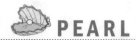 **PEARL**

Often presents in third or fourth grade after a period of absence from school due to illness, vacation or holiday.

REFERENCES

1. Behrman R, Kliegman R, Jenson H: Nelson Textbook of Pediatrics, 17th edition, Philadelphia, W.B. Saunders, 2003.

2. McMillan J, DeAngelis C, Feigin R, Warshaw J: Oski's Pediatrics—Principles and Practice, 3rd edition, Philadelphia, Lippincott, Williams & Wilkins, 1999.

3. Rudolph C, Rudolph A, Hostetter M, Lister G, Siegel N: Rudolph's Pediatrics, 21st edition, New York, McGraw-Hill, 2002.

PULMONARY

Cystic Fibrosis

Inheritance
- Autosomal recessive

Etiology
- Mutation of cystic fibrosis transmembrane conductance regulator
- Most common defect is delta F508

Birth History
- Most common presentation is **meconium ileus**

RADIOLOGIC FINDINGS
- X-ray: calcification in abdomen/scrotum/inguinal canal
- Barium enema: inspissated meconium pellets

Manifestations
- **Nasal polyps**
- Recurrent sinopulmonary infections
- Failure to thrive
- Malabsorption
- **Rectal prolapse**/diarrhea (bulky/foul smelling)
- Bronchiectasis
- Pancreatic insufficiency
- Delayed sexual development
- Clubbing

Diagnosis
Clinical features, or
Abnormal newborn screen, or
Sibling with cystic fibrosis
And
Two elevated sweat chloride tests (> 60 mEq/L), or
Identification of two cystic fibrosis mutations, or
An abnormal nasal potential difference measurement

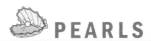

PEARLS

Any child with a nasal polyp should have a sweat chloride test done to rule out cystic fibrosis.

Question may discuss sterile male with atresia or absence of vas deferens.

Cystic Fibrosis

Infections

INFANTS
- *S. aureus*
- Nontypeable *H. influenzae*
- Gram-negative bacilli

CHILDREN AND YOUNG ADULTS
- **P. aeruginosa**

Treatment

- Chest physical therapy
- Bronchodilators
- Inhaled steroids
- DNase—breaks down DNA in thick mucus
- Vitamins/enzyme replacement
- 14 to 21 days of IV antibiotics (aminoglycoside and semisynthetic penicillin) for pulmonary infections

Complications

- Hemoptysis
- Pneumothorax
- Pulmonary hypertension
- Right-sided heart failure

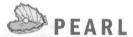

PEARL

Patients are at risk of complications of all fat-soluble vitamin deficiencies (vitamin A, D, E and K) if appropriate nutritional supplements are not taken.

REFERENCES

1. Behrman R, Kliegman R, Jenson H: Nelson Textbook of Pediatrics, 17th edition, Philadelphia, W.B. Saunders, 2003.

2. Rudolph C, Rudolph A, Hostetter M, Lister G, Siegel N: Rudolph's Pediatrics, 21st edition, New York, McGraw-Hill, 2002.

RHEUMATOLOGY

Henoch-Schönlein Purpura

Etiology
- Immunologic vasculitis
- Occurs after viral or group A streptococcal URI

Manifestations

GASTROINTESTINAL
- **Colicky abdominal pain**
- Vomiting
- Upper/lower GI bleeding
- Intussusception

DERMATOLOGIC
- **Purpura without thrombocytopenia**
- Maculopapular **rash on buttocks/lower extremities**

MUSCULOSKELETAL
- Arthritis

RENAL
- Glomerulonephritis
- Nephrotic syndrome

CENTRAL NERVOUS SYSTEM
- Seizures

Treatment
- Supportive
- Corticosteroids for
  - Nephritis
  - Intussusception
  - CNS disease
  - Intestinal hemorrhage

Prognosis
- Excellent; self-resolving in 4 to 6 weeks

Miscellaneous Disorders

BEHCET'S SYNDROME

- Recurrent **oral ulcers, genital ulcers and iritis/uveitis**
- Associated with HLA-B5
- Also can have arthritis and GI symptoms

DERMATOMYOSITIS

- Insidious onset
- Heliotropic erythema (**violaceous rash on eyelids**)
- **Gottron papules**—pale/red hypertrophic skin over metacarpal/interphalangeal joints
- Proximal muscle weakness
- Nailbed telangiectasias
- Elevated creatine kinase
- Treatment: corticosteroids, immunosuppressive agents

SJÖGREN'S SYNDROME

- Burning/itching of eyes
- Dry mouth/eyes
- **Antibodies to La (SSB) and Ro (SSA)**
- Treatment: artificial tears; may need corticosteroids/immunosuppressive agents

Neonatal Systemic Lupus Erythematosus (SLE)

Etiology

MATERNAL ANTINUCLEAR ANTIBODIES
- Transplacental passage to fetus
- Anti-Ro (SSA)
- Anti-La (SSB)

Manifestations

CARDIAC
- Congenital heart block **(permanent)**
- Pericarditis

DERMATOLOGIC
- Scaly erythematous rash of face/trunk/upper extremities

HEMATOLOGIC
- Leukopenia
- Thrombocytopenia
- Anemia

ABDOMINAL
- Hepatosplenomegaly

Treatment

- Supportive
- Corticosteroids
- Cardiac pacing for heart block

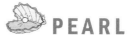

PEARL

Most manifestations resolve except heart block.

Systemic Lupus Erythematosus

Epidemiology
- Females affected much more often than males
- Occurs in late childhood/adolescence
- Increased in Black, Native, Latin and Asian Americans

Diagnosis

CLINICAL DIAGNOSIS (**NEED FOUR OF THE FOLLOWING**)
- Serositis (pleuritis or pericarditis)
- Oral ulcers
- Arthritis
- Photosensitivity
- Hematologic abnormalities (anemia, thrombocytopenia and leukopenia)
- Positive ANA
- CNS symptoms (seizures, psychosis)
- **"Butterfly" malar rash**
- Discoid lupus
- Antibodies
  - Double-stranded DNA
  - **Smith nuclear antigen**
  - Positive LE preparation
  - False-positive serologic test for syphilis
- Renal disease

Labs
- Hypocomplementemia (**low C3,C4 and CH50**)

Complications
- Renal failure
- Infections
- Hypertension
- Increased clotting secondary to "lupus anticoagulant"

Treatment
- Anti-inflammatory (oral steroids, cyclophosphamide)

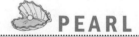

PEARL

A positive ANA occurs in more than 90% of cases (sensitive but not specific).

Juvenile Rheumatoid Arthritis (JRA)

Epidemiology

- Females affected more than males
- Usually presents between 1 and 3 years old
- May also present in late childhood/adolescence

Risk Factor

- **HLA B-27 (pauciarticular)**

Manifestations

- **Morning stiffness**
- Difficulty walking
- **Spiking fevers**
- Hepatosplenomegaly (systemic JRA)
- Lymphadenopathy (systemic JRA)
- Salmon-colored morbilliform rash (systemic JRA)

Diagnosis

DIAGNOSTIC CRITERIA
- Age of onset $<$ 16 years
- Arthritis $\geq$ one joint
- Arthritis $>$ 6 weeks
- Onset type defined in first 6 months
  - Polyarticular: $\geq$ five joints
  - Pauciarticular $\leq$ four joints
  - Systemic—arthritis and fever
- Exclusion of other forms of arthritis

Labs

- Anemia
- Leukocytosis
- Thrombocytosis
- High ESR

Treatment

- NSAIDS (initial treatment)
- Anti-inflammatory (oral steroids, immunosuppressives)
- Physical therapy

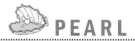

PEARL

JRA has arthritis with anemia, thrombocytosis and leukocytosis, whereas SLE has arthritis with pancytopenia.

Prognosis of Juvenile Rheumatoid Arthritis

POLYARTICULAR

RF positive: Poor (especially with older age of onset)
ANA positive: Good

PAUCIARTICULAR

ANA positive: Excellent (except eyes)
RF positive: Poor
HLA B-27:   Good

SYSTEMIC

Pauciarticular: Good
Polyarticular: Poor

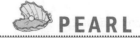

PEARL

Girls with pauciarticular arthritis, early onset disease (< 6 years old) with a positive ANA have increased risk of developing **chronic uveitis.**

Classification of Juvenile Rheumatoid Arthritis	POLYARTICULAR	PAUCIARTICULAR	SYSTEMIC
Cases	40-50%	40-50%	10-20%
No. of Joint	≥ 5 symmetric	≤ 4 (can be one joint)	Variable
Joints	Knees Elbows Ankles Wrists Cervical	Knees Ankles	All joints
Fevers	Yes	No	Yes
Iridocyclitis/uveitis	Rare	**Common (high with + ANA)**	Rare
ANA	50%	80%	10%
Rheumatoid factor	10%	Rare	Rare

REFERENCES

1. Behrman R, Kliegman R, Jenson H: Nelson Textbook of Pediatrics, 17th edition, Philadelphia, W.B. Saunders, 2003.

2. Shah B, Laude T: Atlas of Pediatric Clinical Diagnosis, 1st edition, Philadelphia, W.B. Saunders, 2000.

3. Cassidy J, Petty R: Textbook of Pediatric Rheumatology, 4th edition, Philadelphia, W.B. Saunders, 2001.

4. McMillan J, DeAngelis C, Feigin R, Warshaw J: Oski's Pediatrics—Principles and Practice, 3rd edition, Philadelphia, Lippincott, Williams & Wilkins, 1999.

STATISTICS

Basic Statistics

	DISEASE PRESENT	NO DISEASE
Positive Test	a	b
Negative Test	c	d

Sensitivity: $a / (a + c)$
Specificity: $d / (b + d)$
Positive predictive value: $a / (a + b)$
Negative predictive value: $d / (c + d)$
Prevalence: $(a + c) / (a + b + c + d)$
False negative: $c / (a + c)$
False positive: $b / (b + d)$

Basic Statistics

	DISEASE DEVELOPS	NO DISEASE
Exposure	a	b
No Exposure	c	d

Relative risk: $\dfrac{a / (a + b)}{c / (c + d)}$

Odds ratio: ad / bc

Alpha error: A false-positive error. Alpha is the probability of saying that there is a difference between treatments when there is not.

Beta error: A false-negative error. Beta is the probability of saying that there is no difference between treatments when there is one.

Power: 1—Beta

Confidence interval: Statistical precision of an observed effect. If confidence intervals of relative risk include 1.0, the results are *not statistically significant.*

Study Designs

CASE CONTROL STUDY

- Retrospective observational study
- Cases (with disease) and controls (without disease)
- Calculates an **odds ratio**
- Used for *rare diseases*
- Subject to recall bias and survivorship bias

COHORT STUDY

- Prospective observational study
- Cohort and controls followed over time to see if disease develops
- Calculate a **relative risk**
- Used for *rare exposures*

CLINICAL TRIAL

- Prospective experimental study
- Treatment group and controls
- Usually randomized and double-blinded
- *Highest quality study*

CROSS-SECTIONAL SURVEY

- Survey of population at *a single point in time*
- Estimate disease prevalence

Bias

RECALL BIAS

- Due to error of memory of participants
- Occurs in case-control studies

LEAD-TIME BIAS

- Occurs when disease diagnosed earlier owing to screening
- Survival appears to be prolonged but is not
- Time between diagnosis and death is prolonged

OBSERVATIONAL BIAS

- Responses of study participants or observers are subjective based on arm of study
- Occurs in unblinded studies

LENGTH BIAS

- Screening test will detect large numbers of *slowly* progressive diseases and miss the rapid spreading ones
- Causes overestimation of screening test effectiveness

REFERENCES

1. Behrman R, Kliegman R, Jenson H: Nelson Textbook of Pediatrics, 17th edition, Philadelphia, W.B. Saunders, 2003.

2. Fletcher R, Fletcher S, Wagner E: Clinical Epidemiology—The Essentials. 3rd edition, Baltimore, Williams & Wilkins, 1996.

SURGERY

Acute Abdominal Pain

ETIOLOGY	DIAGNOSTIC CLUES/COMMENTS

Appendicitis	**Fecalith on radiograph**
	Pain
	    Periumbilical
	    Midepigastric
	    Right lower quadrant

Gastroenteritis	Vomiting/diarrhea
Pneumonia	Patient with coughing/respiratory symptoms Diagnose with **chest radiograph**
Constipation	Left lower quadrant pain Palpable mass
Urinary tract infection	Dysuria
Pancreatitis	Can have **normal amylase** Ultrasound helps diagnose
Peptic ulcer	Epigastric pain (can awaken child) Guaiac-positive stools Diagnose with gastric endoscopy

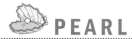 PEARL

Elevated amylase can occur from parotitis, anorexia nervosa, diabetes mellitus or diseases of the salivary gland.

Malrotation

Manifestations

NEWBORN
- **Bilious vomiting**
- Abdominal obstruction/distention
- Often presents within first week

OLDER INFANTS
- Recurrent abdominal pain
- Vomiting

Associations

- **Volvulus—life threatening**

Radiographic Findings

ABDOMINAL X-RAY
- Airless rectum on plain film
- Large gastric bubble

UPPER GI
- **"Bird's beak"**—with volvulus
- **"Corkscrew"**

BARIUM ENEMA
- **Malposition of the cecum**

Treatment

- Nasogastric tube
- IV fluids
- Reduction of volvulus and lysis of Ladd bands

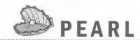

PEARL

Most common cause of **newborn intestinal obstruction.**

Intussusception

Incidence
- 75% occur in children under 2 years of age

Etiology
CHILDREN UNDER 2 YEARS OF AGE
- Usually no lead point found

CHILDREN UNDER 2 YEARS OF AGE
- Lead points are more common
  - **Meckel diverticulum** (most common)
    Typically presents at age 2
    Painless rectal bleeding
    2 feet from ileocecal valve
    Occurs in 2% of population
    2 inches in length
    Lined with gastric mucosa
  - Polyps
  - Foreign body
  - Lymphoma

Manifestations
- **Colicky abdominal pain**
- Child will draw up legs with episodes
- Vomiting
- **Lethargy** between painful episodes

Diagnosis
- Barium enema ("**coiled-spring appearance**")

Treatment
- Barium enema
- Surgery (indicated with failure of enema reduction)

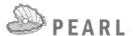 **PEARL**

Examination may find **"sausage-shaped" mass** in right lower quadrant and history may describe **"currant jelly" stools**.

REFERENCES

1. Behrman R, Kliegman R, Jenson H: Nelson Textbook of Pediatrics, 17th edition, Philadelphia, W.B. Saunders, 2003.

2. Rudolph C, Rudolph A, Hostetter M, Lister G, Siegel N: Rudolph's Pediatrics, 21st edition, New York, McGraw-Hill, 2002.

UROLOGY

Urology Pearls

HYPOSPADIAS

- Opening of the urethral meatus is on the ventral surface of the penis.
- Surgery needed for severe cases.
- **Do not circumcise** children with hypospadias (foreskin needed for surgical correction).

CIRCUMCISION

- Not medically necessary or recommended by the AAP
- Decision should be based on *best interest of child*.
- Urinary tract infections are more common in uncircumcised males.
- Recommended in cases in which there is increased risk of UTI (hydronephrosis and reflux).

PARAPHIMOSIS

- Occurs if foreskin is retracted behind coronal sulcus
- Prepuce cannot be pulled back over the glans.
- Treatment: lubrication and manual reduction or surgery

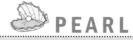 PEARL

An uncircumcised male prepuce becomes fully retractable by the age of 3 years.

Testicle Issues

UNDESCENDED TESTICLES

- After the age of 12 months requires evaluation and referral
- Undescended testicles are at risk for infertility, malignancy and torsion
- Orchiopexy is usually done between 9 to 15 months
- Hormone treatment is infrequently utilized

VARICOCELE

- Abnormal dilatation of the pampiniform plexus
- Usually on left side
- **"Bag of worms"** description
- Decreases with lying down and increases with Valsalva maneuver/standing
- Surgery indicated for large varicoceles, teste size differences or pain in the affected teste

HYDROCELE

- Fluid surrounds testicle
- **Transilluminates**
- Mass does not reach the inguinal ring (noncommunicating)
- Monitor for the first year of life
- Surgery if persists after 1 year

Testicular Pain

EPIDIDYMITIS

- Most common cause of testicular pain in men older than 18 years of age
- Unilateral scrotal pain
- **Cremasteric reflex present**
- May be associated with penile discharge (clear, white or gray)
- In sexually active teenager etiology usually *C. trachomatis or N. gonorrhoeae*
- Painful urination
- Urinalysis reveals sterile pyuria
- Treatment: bed rest and antibiotics

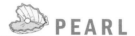

PEARL

Elevation of scrotum may *relieve pain* in epididymitis but worsen pain in testicular torsion.

TORSION OF THE TESTIS

- Most common cause of testicular pain in boys older than 12 years of age
- Rare in boys younger than 10 years of age
- **Cremasteric reflex is nearly always absent**
- Painful, swollen testis (high or retracted)
- **Bell clapper deformity**—inadequate fixation of testis in scrotum
- If pain < 6 hours, attempt manual detorsion
- Surgery is indicated
- Contralateral testis should also be surgically fixed

TORSION OF THE APPENDIX TESTIS

- Most common cause of testicular pain between 2 and 11 years of age
- Rare in adolescence
- Tender mass (3 to 5-mm) on upper pole of testis
- **"Blue dot sign"**
- Surgery is not indicated
- Pain management

REFERENCES

1. Behrman R, Kliegman R, Jenson H: Nelson Textbook of Pediatrics, 17th edition, Philadelphia, W.B. Saunders, 2003.

2. Rudolph C, Rudolph A, Hostetter M, Lister G, Siegel N: Rudolph's Pediatrics, 21st edition, New York, McGraw-Hill, 2002.

Index